Go Diana! This book is an excellent, holi
women of all ages. I found myself encourag
I enjoyed this entertaining and informative
know info on artificial sweeteners, to workout and meal plans, to
"spiritual fitness" help, this book will be a true asset to anyone's
life.

—REBECCA ST JAMES
AWARD-WINNING RECORDING ARTIST

Everything you need to know about diet and nutrition founded
in true wisdom.

—SHANDI FINNESSEY
MISS USA 2004
CONTESTANT, *DANCING WITH THE STARS* (SEASON 4)

Juggling eating right, getting adequate exercise, and staying spiritually fit can be a challenge for any woman. *Fit for Faith* is an
excellent guide to motivate and encourage those who are ready
to experience a healthier lifestyle and a genuine acceptance of
God's beautiful design. Diana Anderson shares not only her
helpful instructions on proper diet and exercise routines, but also
inspiring spiritual truths that will resonate within every reader.

—HEATHER SCHULTZ
FOUNDER, THE PINK DRESS MINISTRY
AUTHOR, *A HAPPIER YOU*

Diana is a young woman after God's own heart whose smile is
as charming as her wit. She takes her life's experiences and gives
young women tangible tools and insight that can help them be
successful in both their faith and fitness journeys. She has the
ability to positively influence others to live for Christ, especially
in the realm of keeping our minds, bodies and spirits in shape.
She has true passion for the Lord, for people and for fitness.

—MICHELLE PENA
CO-OWNER, PREMIER FITNESS
FITNESS BUSINESS CONSULTANT AND CO-FOUNDER OF TWELVE SPOT
MINISTRIES, TYLER, TEXAS

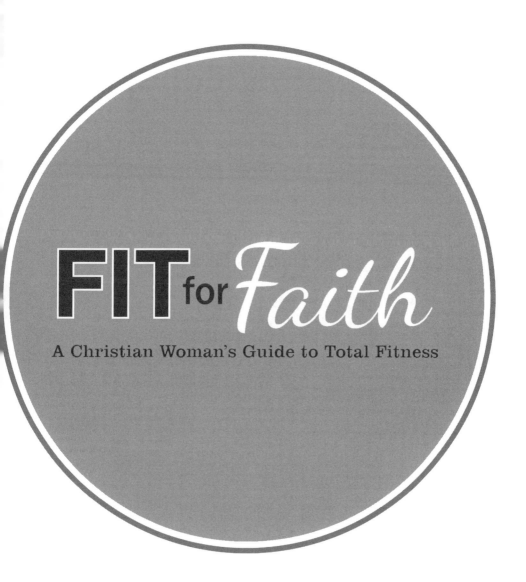

FIT for *Faith*

A Christian Woman's Guide to Total Fitness

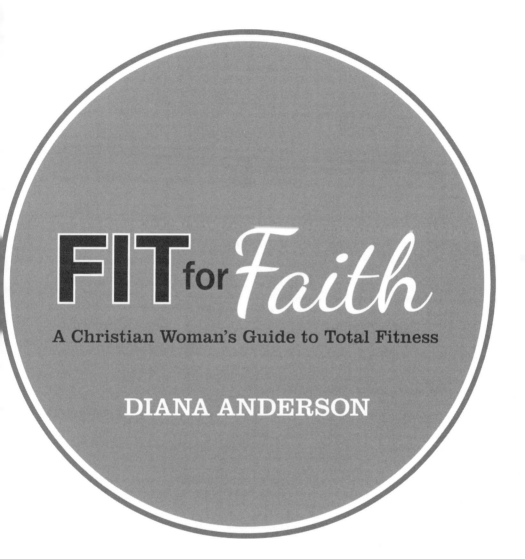

FIT for *Faith*

A Christian Woman's Guide to Total Fitness

DIANA ANDERSON

CREATION
HOUSE

FIT FOR FAITH by Diana Anderson
Published by Creation House
A Charisma Media Company
600 Rinehart Road
Lake Mary, Florida 32746
www.charismamedia.com

Photographs courtesy of Carly Sharawi and Premier Fitness of Tyler, Texas.

Design Director: Bill Johnson
Cover design by Nancy Panaccione

Visit the author's Web sites: www.dianafit.com and www.facebook.com/dianaandersoninc

Library of Congress Control Number: 2011932335
International Standard Book Number: 978-1-61638-620-7

This book contains the opinions and ideas of its author. It is solely for informational and educational purposes and should not be regarded as a substitute for professional medical treatment. The nature of your body's health condition is complex and unique. Therefore, you should consult a health professional before you begin any new exercise, nutrition, or supplementation program or if you have questions about your health. Neither the author nor the publisher shall be liable or responsible for any loss or damage allegedly arising from any information or suggestion in this book.

The statements in this book about consumable products or food have not been evaluated by the Food and Drug Administration. The publisher is not responsible for your specific health or allergy needs that may require medical supervision. The publisher is not responsible for any adverse reactions to the consumption of food or products that have been suggested in this book.

First edition

11 12 13 14 15 — 9 8 7 6 5 4 3 2 1
Printed in Canada

DEDICATION

First and foremost, I dedicate this book to my great God and Savior, Jesus Christ. He is my Source and my Strength. I live to honor You, Abba.

For the grace of God has appeared that offers salvation to all people. It teaches us to say "No" to ungodliness and worldly passions, and to live self-controlled, upright and godly lives in this present age, while we wait for the blessed hope—the appearing of the glory of our great God and Savior, Jesus Christ, who gave himself for us to redeem us from all wickedness and to purify for himself a people that are his very own, eager to do what is good.

—TITUS 2:11–14

Second, I dedicate this book to my parents, Mitchell and Barbara. Mom, I can't imagine where I'd be without your endless love, care, support, encouragement, and most of all, your prayers. You are the epitome of the "Proverbs 31" woman, and I can only pray I'll be like you when I grow up! Daddy, I can't wait to play tennis, mountain bike, and flex my muscles with you on the golden streets of glory. I'll run strong until I meet you there. Your faith in me blesses me each day.

My son, keep your father's command and do not forsake your mother's teaching. Bind them always on your heart; fasten them around your neck. When you walk, they will guide you; when you sleep, they will watch over you; when you awake, they will speak to you.

—PROVERBS 6:20–22

CONTENTS

INTRODUCTION

I SPENT YEARS OF my life thinking weights were for shot-putters and that healthy eating meant relinquishing pizza in favor of flavorless tofu forever. Despite being involved in sports, I didn't feel energetic, and I certainly didn't look athletic. Long story short, my personal trainer and great friend Michael Prince taught me the numerous advantages of weight lifting—dispelling the myth that dumbbells turn girls into the Hulk—and showed me that eating healthfully is essential to a fit lifestyle.

Near the end of my battle with an eating disorder I, as a three-part being comprised of a spirit, soul, and body, came to see that the Lord cares very much about my physical health (1 Thess. 5:23). God's Word says, "Do you not know that your bodies are temples of the Holy Spirit, who is in you, whom you have received from God? You are not your own; you were bought at a price. Therefore glorify God with your bodies" (1 Cor. 6:19–20).

By looking to exercise for control and food for comfort, I had allowed the light of God to be snuffed out in my life. I had placed my obsession on a pedestal and exalted my self over the Spirit in me. I now know that the Lord desires that we treat these temples of flesh and blood with respect and godliness. That doesn't mean we can never take a vacation from the gym or have a cheeseburger every once in a while. It simply means that our bodies are meant for much more than satisfying the five senses—they are to be living sacrifices, "holy and acceptable to God"(Rom. 12:1).

Since I began working out and eating right seven years ago, I have seen my body undergo amazing transformations inside and out. Not only am I toned, trim, and strong, but I have tons of energy, less stress, and one heck of an immune system. I sleep like a baby, I focus better while working, and I'm more revved up and confident to serve God! You see, being in shape does more than just improve our appearance and ward off osteoporosis; it enhances our self-esteem and helps us feel empowered, prepared, and capable to face the capriciousness of life, whether on the mission field, in the office, or at the dinner table.

This is my second fitness book. Since writing *Miss University* for young college women, I have continued to enjoy and appreciate the value of exercise and healthy eating as they relate to my spirit and my walk with God. It amazes me how timeless and relevant the Bible is from beginning to end. Whatever our question, concern, or care, the Word has a remedy in its pages. In the last few years I have implemented biblical truths pertaining to diet, sickness, oppression, and even simple rest and have experienced life-changing results. Just as I was eager to help young women get fired up about fitness, I am thrilled to rekindle those flames as we delve into God's Word and get fit for faith!

Oh, and don't forget your workout gear. You're gonna need it!

1

MISS UNIVERSITY GRADUATES

A Time of Transition

AS THE NAME of this chapter implies, I am now a college graduate. I earned my degree in radio-TV-film and am now a film critic/highly educated moviegoer. I'm also scribbling down scenes in various screenplays I've begun, but I find myself coming back to this whole fitness business! Training women and educating them about "faithful" workouts and nutrition is an absolute joy and privilege. Maybe I should write a screenplay about a coed who, despite dangerous adversaries like unwholesome cafeteria food, late-night studying, and a taxing schedule, manages to graduate stronger and fitter than ever! Something tells me that wouldn't translate into riveting action on the big screen.

Although the premise I just pitched for you would never help Reese Witherspoon win her next Oscar, it is my 100 percent true story, which I feel compelled to share with you. In *Miss University*, Michael and I laid a solid foundation for creating and maintaining a healthy lifestyle throughout high school and college. And though there are myriad other fitness regimens and programs continually propagated from bookshelves, magazine racks, and infomercials, the message we presented possesses one unique difference that still separates it from the rest. That difference is purpose.

Perhaps you are familiar with Rick Warren's best-selling book *The Purpose-Driven Life*. In it he writes, "The purpose of your life is far greater than your own personal fulfillment, your peace of mind, or even your happiness. . . . If you want to know why you were placed on this planet, you must begin with God. You were born by his purpose and for his purpose."[1]

So what does working out have to do with a life lived purposefully for the Lord? If we believe that our bodies are temples of the Holy Spirit and that we are to glorify God with them, then the answer is clear. Our lives are comprised of thoughts, beliefs, attitudes, behaviors, and actions. Leading a healthy lifestyle is a daily action that strengthens us for our spiritual calling and occupation, and it is scientifically proven to positively affect our thoughts and attitudes. While the world may emphasize diet and exercise as a means to achieve a clean bill of health and a decent physique, as Christians we see that the purpose of fitness is far greater than temporal results and the superficial significance we place upon it. Put quite simply, being healthy helps our purpose.

Working out and eating right were vital parts of my life for half of my high school years and throughout my college career. I succeeded academically without stressing out, gaining weight, or losing focus. And as I stand on the threshold of a bright new chapter, I know that same commitment to fitness will enable me to navigate life's opportunities, weather the storms, and remain anchored to the Rock of Ages. The foundation I laid continues to be augmented as I learn new exercises, implement fresh routines, discover healthy foods, and obey the Shepherd's voice—the building blocks of fitness.

With this book I wish to share with you some of the things the Lord has taught me through His Word as I have sought it for direction, encouragement, explanation, and revelation. The Word of God truly is "living and active," as it says in the Book of Hebrews, and is unequivocally the finest resource we have for living a fruitful, healthful life.

As I said in the introduction, don't leave your weight-lifting gloves and tennis shoes at the door. This is a contact book! I mentioned a few moments ago that two of the building blocks of fitness are new exercises and fresh routines. Today, women seem to be busier than ever, and our hectic schedules often relegate working out to the optional part of the daily to-do list. Careers, families, social activities, and excuses are all challenges faced by women who seek to make fitness a priority.

Over the last two years I have incorporated circuit training into my routine as a way to train efficiently, providing an incredible, calorie-blasting workout in very little time. Another glorious revelation I've embraced is that I can get an awesome workout without ever leaving my house! With very little—or zero—equipment, you can transform your living room into your own personal training studio. Who needs a gym membership? I've also learned that working out with other women is a terrific way to keep motivated and stay committed. With new workouts you can do anywhere in no time and friends to cheer you on and pump you up, you'll be feeling (and looking!) even more fit and fabulous.

I pray that this book is a blessing to you. It's my prayer that the Holy Spirit speaks to you and helps you find within these pages a truth you've never heard before, an answer you've been looking for, an encouragement you needed to hear, or even diet advice or a few new workouts to keep you on track and on your toes. Now, go grab a cup of green tea and prepare to be fit for faith!

2

A TIME TO EVERY PURPOSE

Glorifying God in All We Do

So whether you eat or drink or whatever you do, do it all for the glory of God.
—1 Corinthians 10:31

To most of us, glorifying God in everything we do may sound like an exaggeration if not an impossibility. Are we expected to turn off iTunes and sing hymns all day? Should we get off Facebook and stay glued to the Good Book? Are we to protest movies and host all-night prayer meetings?

Certainly praising God, reading His Word, and spending time in prayer are wonderful, invaluable things that bless our Maker and strengthen our spirit, but becoming monks who draw away from modern culture and cling to ascetic seclusion is not what most of us are called to do. We are to be salt and light in the world, not outside it (Matt. 5:13–17). Jesus instructed us to let our lights "shine before men, that they may see your good works and give glory to your Father in heaven" (Matt. 5:16). How can we be lights in darkness if we live in sunshine? How can we keep things fresh and give flavor if we dwell in an untouched, gourmet kitchen?

Faith Fact: In the Old Testament, every animal sacrifice was commanded to be seasoned with salt. Salt symbolizes the righteousness of Christ. So, just as salt makes meat tasty, the righteousness of Christ makes us virtuous.

Fit Fact: It's recommended that we consume 1 teaspoon, or 2,300 milligrams, of salt per day. However, seven out of ten adults in America consume 2.3 times this amount. Studies show that those who eat too much of it increase their risk of heart disease and stroke. To cut back, limit your intake of processed and manufactured foods.[1]

I submit to you that if we consider the uses and importance of salt and light both literally and symbolically, we can begin to apply those principles to our daily lives and realize that we really can give glory to our Father in everything—even working out and eating right.

Let There Be Light!

Light is the first of painters. There is no object so foul that intense light will not make it beautiful.

—Ralph Waldo Emerson[2]

The significance of light and its manifold uses are no mystery to humankind. Without natural sunlight, we wouldn't be able to work or play outdoors, travel, or be able to distinguish day from night. And without Edison's "bright" idea, which helped us obtain light after hours, I wouldn't be able to type this paragraph right now! Light facilitates productivity by brightening our surroundings and provides direction by illuminating our way.

The word *light* is used 309 times in the King James Version of the Bible.[3] Whether functioning through a lighthouse, lamp, flame, candle, or burning bush, light is a common symbol of Christianity used to represent God's manifest presence in the world. First John 1:5 tells us that God is light, and Jesus called Himself the "light of the world" (John 8:12). After Jesus's death and resurrection, the Holy Spirit descended as flaming tongues and rested on each of the believers gathered at Pentecost. This marvelous act signified that the believers were sanctified and filled with the grace of the Holy Ghost.

As believers in Jesus Christ, this holy flame has come to reside within each of us. Jesus proclaimed that He was the light of the world so long as He was on the earth (John 9:5). Now that He sits at the right hand of the Father, we are the world's light source through which the Holy Spirit shines (Matt. 5:14).

You probably sang the song "This Little Light of Mine" in Sunday school when you were a kid. Though the lyrics are simple and the melody is quaint, the message is pure and powerful. The light we have is not to be hidden under a bushel—whatever that is—nor blown out by the enemy; it's to be shone all over the world, from college campuses to distant tribes half a world away "'til Jesus comes"! The only thing I would change in this song is the word *little*. Our light is astronomical in size, more powerful than any Jedi lightsaber, and more brilliant than the gamma-ray bursts seen halfway across the universe. It's the light of the Holy Spirit, the same powerful entity that raised our Savior from the grave!

ENLIGHTENED BY THE HOLY SPIRIT

> Now we have received, not the spirit of the world, but the spirit which is of God; that we might know the things that are freely given to us of God.
>
> —1 CORINTHIANS 2:12, KJV

So just what is this light in us? What is that ineffable spark that the world can't help but notice nor succeed in stifling? The moment we accepted Jesus Christ as our Lord and Savior, we received the Holy Spirit, who, according to Ephesians 1:13, is the seal of our salvation and an identifying factor of our possession of salvation through Him (Rom. 8:9). Entire books have been written and detailed series taught on this third part of our holy and perfect triune God, and I encourage you to read and learn all you can. For the purposes of this chapter, however, I'll explore the ways in which the Spirit helps us glorify God through healthy living. We can't do it without Him!

> But when he, the Spirit of truth, comes, he will guide you into all truth. He will not speak on his own; he will speak only what he hears, and he will tell you what is yet to come.
>
> —JOHN 16:13

One of the primary roles of the Holy Spirit is that of a guide. We can rest assured that the Holy Spirit, as the Spirit *of truth*, always leads us according to what is godly and helps us discern between truth and falsehood. Since He lives inside us, He has direct access to every part of our being, from shallow, selfish thoughts all the way through to our most profound longings and every secret struggle. Like Christ, He is willingly submitted to the Father, so therefore everything we hear from Him is according to God, not to His own initiative.

I can hear you asking me now just how we hear from the Holy Spirit. While I don't discount those who claim to have heard the very voice of God, I don't believe such occurrences are what we should be expecting on a daily basis. Based on the terrified reactions of biblical saints who heard or saw the Lord face-to-face, I believe the Spirit speaks softly within us, because, after all, that's where He lives. All He needs is a heart willing to listen and a mind that is renewed and ready for His counsel.

The Book of Acts records several occasions when the Holy Spirit spoke to Peter and Paul. You may say, "Yeah, but they were men chosen personally by Christ to take the gospel all over the world, and I'm here in Georgia and probably won't ever go on a mission trip." Yes, but that same Spirit that indwelt the early apostles lives in us today. Before His ascension into heaven, Jesus promised that His Father would send the Holy Spirit to be our Helper and abide with us forever (John 14:16). His divide guidance is needed by homemakers, professionals, retirees, and students today just as much as it was by believers two thousand years ago.

Every day consists of one decision after another, from whether to get out of bed at 6:00 a.m. to which pajamas you'll put on at night. Of course, not every choice is as straightforward as starting a new day or as harmless as picking out clothing. But what about fitness? How can the Holy Spirit help us make "true" decisions when it comes to how we eat and exercise?

FIT, FAITHFUL, AND FILLED WITH THE SPIRIT

> But when he, the Spirit of truth, comes, he will guide you into all truth. He will not speak on his own; he will speak only what he hears, and he will tell you what is yet to come.
>
> —JOHN 16:13

I haven't always depended on the Holy Spirit for guidance. It was only near the end of my struggle with anorexia and a binge-eating disorder that I realized God took great interest in the details of my life and wanted me to be well even more than my parents did. For nearly two years I simply reasoned that my problems were silly and mundane, especially when compared to the events unfolding around the world and the needs of sick, hungry, and homeless millions in third-world countries. I prayed only about the things that seemed worthy in my eyes, and working out obsessively and eating excessively hardly seemed to fit into that category. One day while flipping aimlessly through the New Testament, I came upon a passage that suddenly spoke directly to my heart:

Humber yourselves, therefore, under God's mighty hand, that he might lift you up in due time. Cast all your anxiety on him because he cares for you.

—1 PETER 5:6–7

The word *all* seemed to highlight itself on the page. God was encouraging me to lay down every single worry and care before Him, even those concerning caloric intake. As I knelt and cried out to Him, pouring out all my frustrations, fears, and guilt, I truly began to see God as my *Abba*—Daddy. My father recently went to be with the Lord, but I'll never forget how he would stop whatever he was doing, regardless of his schedule, to listen to my problems, offer me advice, or simply ease my worries with one heartfelt hug. Just as he would kneel down to me when I was a little girl to listen intently and wrap me in his arms, so God bends down to hear our cares (Ps. 116:2)!

In the Sermon on the Mount, Jesus instructed us not to be anxious for anything because "your heavenly Father knows that you need all these things" (Matt. 6:32, NKJV). This is just as comforting to me today as it was two years ago when I finally put an end to my self-condemnation and told the enemy to go back to where he came from. At last I realized God had provided me a Helper, a Comforter, a Guide to help me live victoriously in every area of my life, not just the ones I deemed important. Now I know that to God nothing is trivial or insignificant. He even knows how many hairs are on my head (Luke 12:7)!

Though the Holy Spirit had been within me since I accepted Christ in the second grade, I hadn't realized the importance of having a relationship with Him. For the most part I was doing all the right things, doing my best to live a "good, Christian life," but there always seemed to be a puzzle piece missing, a warmth I wasn't feeling. Only by being brought to the end of myself and my own efforts would I find the peace my soul was pining for. First Corinthians 6:19 began echoing against the darkened chambers of my spirit, and I could sense light filtering in. *The Holy Spirit is in me*, I thought. *He's the One who makes me like Christ, not me.*

The morning after I'd cried out to God and emptied my heart of its pent-up burdens, I got out of bed feeling rather triumphant. I meditated on the verses I'd read the night before and began my day by thinking through the temptations I'd face, the pressures I'd feel, and I also thanked God for the victory over them. And each time my flesh was tempted to indulge in food I didn't need or dwell on my weight and my workouts, I spoke to the Holy Spirit: *I have already claimed Christ's power. He has dealt with this! Handle this situation through me.*

Galatians 5:16, which says, "Walk by the Spirit, and you will not carry out the desire of the flesh" (NAS), proved an indispensable truth. The word for "walk" is *peripateo*, which means to "tread all around."[4] "Treading all around" by the Spirit enables us to avoid the moral pitfalls that surround us. Before I trusted the Holy Spirit to guide me, I tried to fight my battles in my own strength by telling myself what not to do. By avoiding certain foods and habits, I focused on them, and by focusing on them, I drifted toward them. The wonderful thing I discovered about walking by the Spirit is that I began to drift toward Him! No longer did I dwell on all the negatives and what I shouldn't do. No longer did I fixate on how many calories I'd expended that day versus how many I'd consumed. By the Spirit, my focus shifted from myself to my Savior. This new perspective made all the difference in how I viewed my body and, consequently, how I treated it.

Today, keeping fit is no longer about me and a carnal desire to be a certain dress size or earn the praises of people. Leading a healthy lifestyle has taken on a deeper, spiritual dimension, one that transcends strength, slimness, muscle tone, and a body fat percentage by supplanting superficial goals with God-glorifying values. As Paul articulately wrote nearly two thousand years ago, "Physical training is good, but training for godliness is much better, promising benefits in this life and in the life to come" (1 Tim. 4:8, NLT). Before I knew God desired a personal, intimate relationship with me through the Holy Spirit, physical training had far surpassed "good" in my life. I had exalted it above godliness and fashioned it into my own idol, which I worshiped and meditated on religiously.

The Holy Spirit has taught me that every decision I make—including the one to lace up my tennis shoes and get to the gym—either brings God glory or it doesn't (1 Cor. 10:31). Allow me to explain: If you had a choice between a bacon cheeseburger and a turkey sandwich on wheat for lunch, which would you choose to positively fuel your body? Clearly the answer is the turkey sandwich, because nutritious foods provide essential vitamins and minerals, supply energy, and build our immune systems. Conversely, the bacon cheeseburger, filled with saturated fat, promotes diseases such as diabetes and hypertension (high blood pressure). Granted, the occasional cheeseburger is absolutely fine, and might I add, human! What I'm addressing is a day-to-day lifestyle that either facilitates or thwarts our Christian walk. Maintaining a diet of primarily healthy, God-made foods enables our bodies, inhabited by the Holy Spirit, to flourish, while a diet composed mainly of processed, fatty, and unhealthy foods sets our bodies up for sickness, disease, and lethargy.

In the same way the decision to eat a turkey sandwich over a bacon cheeseburger ultimately glorifies God, so too does the decision to go for a run instead of watch *The Hills* or lift weights rather than surf the Net. By running, you activate your immune system, strengthen your heart, keep your arteries clear, ward off viral illnesses, and boost your mood. By lifting weights, you increase muscle mass, which burns more calories. You also improve bone density and balance and reduce your risk for chronic diseases. Being sedentary does none of those things. A British study done in 2008 even suggested that an inactive lifestyle diminishes life expectancy by predisposing the body to aging-related illnesses. It also influences the aging process itself![5] Clearly, physical training has value, and the choice to pursue it is a godly one.

While nonbelievers can certainly respect and appreciate the benefits of fitness, their reasons for doing so are limited to the confines of the flesh and temporal results, such as a trim waistline, a completed marathon, or a longer life. As Christians led by the Spirit, our decision to build our muscles, strengthen our hearts and lungs, and fuel them all with nutritious foods corresponds directly with our decision to follow and serve Christ. The same arms and legs that we strengthen with iron dumbbells in the morning are the very tools we use to serve God the rest of the day. The balanced meals we choose supply all the nutrients we need to feel energized, think clearly, work diligently, and live free of sickness so we can be able and active parts of Christ's body, the church. Regarding it with a spiritual perspective, we can see that fitness has eternal implications that far exceed the reflection in the mirror, the numbers on the scale, and the data of a medical record. Being fit helps put our faith in action.

BE SALTY (WITH AND WITHOUT SWEATING)

> You are the salt of the earth. But if the salt loses its saltiness, how can it be made salty again? It is no longer good for anything, except to be thrown out and trampled by men.
>
> —MATTHEW 5:13

The Sermon on the Mount is undoubtedly one of the most well-known portions of Scripture. Apart from its hard-to-miss placement at the beginning of the New Testament, the reason for the sermon's popularity stems from its strikingly clear and profoundly plain teachings. Sitting on an unknown hill outside of Jerusalem, Jesus succinctly described the way of life His followers would come to embrace and aspire to. The sermon contains a valuable metaphor that compares the ubiquitous natural resources of salt and light with intensely spiritual insights. Since we've dealt with light in the previous sections, we'll now turn our attention to an essential compound of sodium and chlorine.

In biblical days, salt was used as:

- A purifying agent (Lev. 2:13)
- A fertilizer ingredient
- A sign of God's covenant with His people (2 Chron. 13:5)
- A preservative
- A seasoning (Job 6:6)
- A form of payment for Roman soldiers

Undeniably, salt was extremely important to Jesus's contemporaries and their way of life. There are myriad ways in which this multifunctional substance relates to our Christian walk; however, to save time (and keep your attention) I'll only illuminate salt's significance in light of Jesus's words.

Most of us are aware that salt cannot lose its ability to season unless it's chemically altered. So what was Christ referring to when He said, "If the salt loses its saltiness"?

In ancient Jewish society, meals were eaten in the upper rooms of homes, such as the one in which Christ and His disciples shared the Last Supper before His crucifixion. The floors of these rooms were constructed of wood overlaid with plaster. In order to harden the plaster and make the floor durable enough to walk on without cracking, or worse, collapsing, salt was added. Only then was the floor suitable to be "trodden under foot of men." Of course, this mixture then ceased to be suitable for the purpose of seasoning or preserving.

Faith Fact: Scripture tells us in Mark 6:3 that Jesus was a *tekton,* or "master craftsman," before He entered into His ministry at age thirty. It can be presumed He probably knew a thing or two about how floors were built![6]

Jesus was illustrating to believers that we cannot be a blessing to others if we are impure. If we mix our saltiness with a contaminating substance, our "flavor" is neutralized. If we blend biblical truths and instructions with men's traditions and worldly philosophy, our attempts to please God are made in vain. Jesus said Himself, "They worship me in vain; their teachings are but rules taught by men" (Mark 7:7).

After spending four years in a public university, I can attest to the fact that secular humanism is on the rise, propagating the notion that human beings are "undesigned, unintended, and responsible for themselves."[7] I have never been more grateful for my strong Christian upbringing than when I sat in class listening to highly intellectual professors with PhDs consistently promoting post-Christian worldviews in which God was no more sovereign than Mickey Mouse and no more relevant than back issues of *OK!* magazine. Harvard University's humanist chaplain Greg Epstein recently wrote a book titled *Good Without God,* which teaches "we can lead good and moral lives without supernaturalism, without higher powers…without God."[8] As Christians, we know we can do nothing without Christ, let alone lead moral lives in our own strength, and yet so many students and young people are subscribing to the lies by opening up their "salt shakers" to contaminating lectures and worldly reasoning (John 15:5).

Many of my Christian friends, unsure of their faith, quickly became skeptical of the things they had been taught by their Christian parents and pastors. They began to dilute biblical righteousness and godly principles by compromising it with the deceitful, albeit sweet-sounding rhetoric of their professors. By blending salt with plaster, they became flavorless as ambassadors of Christ (2 Cor. 5:20). It wasn't long before they were "trampled underfoot" by the doctrines of men.

The apostle Paul warned young Timothy that some believers would give in to false teaching and accept "myths" (2 Tim. 4:4). It is imperative that we guard our hearts and do as the Bereans did, as recorded in Acts 17:11: "They…searched the Scriptures daily to find out whether these things were so" (NKJV). By studying God's Word, we can ensure that we won't be found defenseless against men's trickery (Eph. 4:14).

Needless to say in a nation in which nativity scenes are viewed as offensive and "Merry Christmas" is becoming a forbidden expression, our society is ready to attack us for our faith. Paul told us persecution would come if we lived godly lives in Christ (2 Tim. 3:12). But don't be intimidated by the flowery language that emanates from academia or silenced by the syrupy New Age gobbledygook gurus and humanists embrace; the Bible tells us we are "more than conquerors" and that nothing can separate us from the love of Christ (Rom. 8:37).

The truth is that adversity is a good indication that you are effectively living out your faith! If no one ever questioned, challenged, or rebuked you for what you believe, it would mean you've become too comfortable in the world—you've lost your flavor, and your light is faint. Peter said we are blessed when we are insulted for the name of Christ (1 Pet. 4:14). Believe me, people—even your friends—may find it silly that you work out primarily to be a healthy, active part of a greater body, i.e., the body of Christ. But don't lose heart; the salt you're shaking might be just the dash of truth they need to lead them toward a relationship with Christ or a revelation of His purpose for their lives.

James said it best, "Consider it pure joy…whenever you face trials of many kinds, because you know that the testing of your faith develops perseverance.…Blessed is the man who perseveres under trial, because when he has stood the test, he will receive the crown of life that God has promised to those who love him" (James 1:2–3, 12).

Fit Fact: Our muscles, much like spiritual perseverance, grow only after undergoing intense exercise in which muscle fibers experience trauma, referred to as muscle injury or damage. Don't worry if you don't see muscle development right away. Muscles immediately begin to adapt to the stress of resistance, but the growth typically takes weeks to be visible. The next time you hit the weights in the gym or resistance in life, you will be stronger!

3

CHEZ YAHWEH

What Would God's Restaurant Be Cookin'?

*Say to the Israelites: "Of all the animals that live on
land, these are the ones you may eat…"*
—Leviticus 11:2

I
T'S RARE TO stroll through the health-and-fitness section of your local
bookstore nowadays without noticing the overflow of diet books proclaiming the newest trimming trend. Atkins and South Beach were only
the beginning. Currently top-selling diet books tout special cookies, lemonade,
apple cider vinegar, and grapefruit as holding the secrets to slim-down success.
Others guarantee a way to drop a significant number of pounds in less than
one week through extreme "cleansing."

While these plans sound absurd, I don't question their effectiveness, at least
for the short term. However, you and I know a balanced diet that includes all
food groups and enjoys indulgences in moderation is the key for maintaining a
healthy weight. But what does the Bible have to say about the foods we eat? Does
God really care as long as we aren't gluttonous? After reading this chapter, perhaps you won't be surprised one day to see two ancient Old Testament books
shelved beside the latest diet crazes.

Fit Fact: "The Centers for Disease Control and Prevention (CDC) estimate
that at any given time, two-thirds of all American adults are on a diet to
either lose weight or prevent weight gain. Of those, 29 percent are men and
44 percent are women. *Yet, only 5 percent of these dieters will be successful
at keeping the lost weight off.*"[1]

DEUTERONOMY AND LEVITICUS—DIET BOOKS?

The first five books of the Old Testament, known as the Torah, which means "instruction" in Hebrew, contain the laws and commandments to which religious Jews adhere. In his book *To Be a Jew*, Rabbi Hayim Halevy Donin writes that the dietary laws found in Leviticus and Deuteronomy are a call to holiness for the Jewish people.[2]

You may be familiar with the term *kosher*, meaning "proper" or "correct," used to describe foods that fit Jewish standards for consumption. Here are a few of the general rules:

- All fruits and vegetables must be inspected for bugs.

- All blood must be drained from meat and poultry or broiled out of it before it is eaten.

- Of the animals allowed to be eaten, the birds and mammals must be slaughtered in accordance with Jewish law.

- Meat cannot be eaten with dairy.

I'm sure many of you are thinking, "OK, but I'm not a Jew. What do their three-thousand-year-old laws have to do with me when I've got the USDA?" Read on, sister.

Faith Fact: The Jewish laws regarding kosher slaughter are so sanitary that kosher butchers and slaughterhouses have been exempted from many USDA regulations.

THE TWO GREAT LAWS

Before we go further, it's important to understand that God gave the Israelites two types of law to abide by after He led them out of Egyptian bondage: the Ten Commandments, which He wrote with His own finger upon stone, and the ordinances and ceremonial rites Moses heard on Mount Sinai and recorded on scrolls.

The Ten Commandments, also known as the moral law and the Decalogue, and the Mosaic Law, comprising the social, moral, and ceremonial commands, are linked in that the commandments define sin and demand the remedies offered by the ceremonial law or ordinances.

For example, in 1,000 B.C., if Ahab coveted Elihu's donkey, he would only have to hear or read the Ten Commandments to know he'd broken God's law. To atone for his sin, he would be required to seek out a spotless female goat, take it to the place of burnt offerings, lay his hands on it to symbolically transfer his sins to the animal, and then slaughter it. But because Jesus Christ became our sacrificial lamb, we no longer are under such laws "but under grace" (Rom. 6:14). Hallelujah!

You see, all those laws and rituals were pictures of man's surrender to the person of God as well as shadows of the ultimate sacrifice to come, which would redeem mankind by eradicating our sins completely, not merely covering them, as the blood of animals did. That sacrifice was made by Jesus Christ in A.D. 33. When He bowed His head and cried, "It is finished," from the cross, God's mighty, unseen hand tore the temple veil in two from top to bottom. This supernatural act after the death of our Savior signified that the ceremonial law system was nailed to the cross (Col. 2:14). Today, when we sin, we confess and repent, knowing we've been forgiven by God's grace.

> Therefore, there is now no condemnation for those who are in Christ Jesus, because through Christ Jesus the law of the Spirit of life set me free from the law of sin and death. For what the law was powerless to do in that it was weakened by the sinful nature, God did by sending his own Son in the likeness of sinful man to be a sin offering. And so he condemned sin in sinful man, in order that the righteous requirements of the law might be fully met in us, who do not live according to the sinful nature but according to the Spirit.
> —ROMANS 8:1–4

New Testament passages like the one above make it abundantly clear that we are no longer under the yoke of the Old Testament laws. However, this doesn't give us free rein to build a shrine for the *Twilight* cast, murder our *frenemies*, or steal mascara. Jesus said that if we love Him, we will keep His commandments (John 14:15). The Ten Commandments made us aware of our sin nature and unrighteousness before we were born again; it was the mirror that showed us our filthiness before a holy God. But that mirror couldn't give us a makeover;

only Jesus's sacrifice could. If we properly understand and appreciate God's gift of grace, our liberty leads us to please Him, seek His will, and keep His commandments as we selflessly serve and love others as He loves us.

JUST FOR THE HEALTH OF IT

Even though Christians aren't bound to the Levitical dietary laws God prescribed for His people under the old covenant, we can certainly apply their principles to our everyday lives and reap extraordinary benefits. It's not a matter of breaking the Law but establishing great health. After all, the author of this diet is the Creator Himself! If He could intelligently design the cosmos, He can most definitely enlighten man with nutritional guidelines.

Fit Fact: God's hygiene laws for Israel are in no way old school or archaic. In fact, hospitals to this day follow nearly every guideline that God laid out originally in the Bible.

Let's remember that each rule and law God gave to Moses was purposeful. Everything from temple rituals to animal sacrifices was rife with symbolism for the nation of Israel and replete with meaning for Christians today who realize those traditions were mere shadows of "things…to come…the reality, however, is found in Christ" (Col. 2:17). Just as there is nothing arbitrary about why the Lord required the Israelites to obey His commands, there is nothing random or insignificant about the food He encouraged or forbade them to eat. The dietary laws were given to provide God's children with excellent health.

SAVE PORKY PIG

Most of you are aware that pork products are off-limits to practicing Jews. But why? What's so terrible about a Christmas ham or pigs in a blanket on a Monday morning? As we examine the reasons for God's dietary decree, we'll find that He was well ahead of twenty-first-century science. Surprise, surprise.

Leviticus 11:3 makes it clear that animals with split hooves that chew the cud (regurgitated food) may be eaten. Pigs, though they have split hooves, do not re-chew their food. Similarly, cud-chewing camels are omitted from our menu because their hooves are undivided. The reason pigs do not re-chew their food is due to their limited anatomy. They, unlike cattle, only have one stomach available to process and refine its contents. Their simply made stomachs and excretory systems were not designed to cleanse themselves of all the putrid and polluted matter entering into them. In other words, when we eat barbecued ribs, we are actually consuming more than we realize. Pigs are the antithesis of picky eaters; they'll eat anything they can get their snouts on, from a fellow swine's droppings to dead, diseased animals.

Besides their toxic diets, pigs also possess large amounts of sulfur in their connective tissues, which can lead to increased blood acidity and osteoporosis. Research has even found that 56 percent of all pork samples are contaminated with salmonella![3] I don't know about you, but I think I'll switch to turkey bacon.

Animals OK for consumption—a.k.a., that chew their cud and have split hooves—include cows, buffalo, goats, sheep, and so forth. These vegetarian critters, whose diets consist of grasses and hay, use their secondary stomachs to thoroughly digest food and eliminate waste. Grass-fed versions of these meat sources have been found to have substantially less fat than their grain-fed counterparts. Not only is grass-fed better for you, it's much tastier.

Fit Fact: Meat and poultry are excellent sources of many important nutrients, such as iron, zinc, vitamin D, magnesium, and B vitamins.

No More Scavenger Hunts!

In Leviticus 11:10 God steers us away from "abominable" fish. (This sounds severe!) In a clamshell, any fish without fins or scales is off-limits. This list consists of shellfish, snails, crabs, shrimp, and lobster. When I first learned this, I wanted to cover my ears, because I cherished ordering shrimp cocktail as an appetizer on special occasions. However, my disappointment soon faded when I heard why the little crustaceans are so offensive.

Finless, scaleless fish are bottom-feeders. They spend their time moseying along the lake or ocean floor, having their fill of fish waste. Due to their physiology, whatever these creatures consume moves directly into their system. This is why scientists can determine water pollution by checking the flesh of shellfish and crustaceans. In essence, these organisms are trash collectors, the marine equivalent of slop-wallowing swine.

Fish with fins and scales, however, are fantastic for us. Tuna, salmon, trout, and halibut are all rich sources of proteins, vitamins, minerals, and essential omega-3 fatty acids, which are proven to stimulate blood circulation, reduce blood pressure, and prevent cancer, to name a few of their benefits.

When buying fish, be sure and shop only for wild-caught brands. The farm-raised variety are more likely to harbor contaminates and lack nutrients.

Fit Fact: In January 2004, the journal *Science* warned that farm-raised salmon contain ten times more toxins than wild salmon.[4]

OUR FEATHERED FRIENDS

Flamingos, pelicans, parrots, penguins! None of these are eligible entrees, but it's not because of their beauty or cuteness.

God included eagles, vultures, owls, and many others among the dirty birds listed in Leviticus 11:13–20. Birds like the previous three are all predators. They feast on the flesh of dead animals and are therefore likely to carry harmful toxins and diseases. Clean birds will have all of the following characteristics:

- Not a bird of prey
- Catch food in the air but bring it to the ground to divide it with their bills, if possible, before eating
- Must spread their toes so that three front toes are on one side of a perch and the hind toe on the other side
- Must have craws or crops (stomach-like pouches used for digestion)
- They must have an elongated middle front toe and a hind toe
- Must have a gizzard with a double lining that can easily be separated

We can deduce from this list that most wading and aquatic birds are unclean. It's just as well in my opinion. They're just too darn pretty!

The Creepy Crawlies

I know it's difficult to pass up the temptation to snack on dirt daubers and bees on the jogging trail, but it's a good thing you do. Leviticus 11:20 tells us that all "winged creeping things" (ASV) that can also walk on all fours "are to be detestable to you" (NIV). As if they weren't already?

Faith Fact: If you're smarter than a fifth grader, you know insects have six legs. So why does the Bible use the word *four* when describing creeping things? This discrepancy is another indication that the numbers of the Old Testament are not to be taken literally. Why? For the simple reason that Moses was writing to accommodate God's instruction to the common practice rather than assert a strict, literal description. Analogous to this is many people's incorrect usage of *bug* to describe spiders, millipedes, and centipedes.

Believe it or not, the insects the Bible permits us to eat, i.e., crickets and grasshoppers, are rich protein sources and also contain iron, calcium, phosphorus, and vitamins. An added bonus, they don't require cooking!

Faith Fact: John the Baptist subsisted by eating locusts and wild honey while living in the wilderness, making "straight the way of the Lord" (John 1:23).

I hope none of you are accustomed to eating salamander salads. Reptiles and amphibians are on the do not eat list as well. Leviticus 11:31 says that animals that move along the ground are unfit to eat. Not having cloven hooves and not being cud-chewers doubly disqualifies the croaking and slithering from being dietary staples. I'm not complaining!

The Laws on Paws

My miniature schnauzers, Dug and Dora, can sleep soundly because dogs and cats are for fetching and lap-laying only! Leviticus 11:27 says that animals that walk on paws are not to be eaten. Other unclean critters include skunks, raccoons, squirrels, as well as lions and tigers and bears—oh my! Can you imagine seeing a skunk sandwich on the Subway menu or squirrel soup at Applebee's?

Fit Fact: Raccoons, squirrels, pigs, bears, and other off-limits animals are known carriers of diseases such as trichinosis, which is caused by parasites that can infect and damage many body tissues.

THE WISEST MAN IN THE WORLD SPEAKS OUT ON REFINED CARBS!

In case you didn't know, King Solomon (King David's son) was not only exceedingly wealthy and successful in making Israel a flourishing nation, but he was also blessed with abundant wisdom. First Kings 4:29–31 tells us that the breadth of his understanding was as measureless as the sand on the beach!

Most of us are familiar with Solomon's well-known proverbs, such as, "Trust in the LORD with all your heart and lean not on your own understanding; in all your ways acknowledge him, and he will make your paths straight" (Prov. 3:5–6). The Bible says that kings from all over the world traveled to Jerusalem to hear the sensible sayings of Israel's king.

The topics of his insightful speeches ranged from discipline and diligence to gluttony and greed. Regarding gluttony, we read, "Don't associate with those who drink too much wine, or with those who gorge themselves on meat" (Prov. 23:20, hcsb). Solomon was even inspired to talk about refined carbohydrates. Don't believe me? Here's proof:

> If you find honey, eat only what you need…It is not good to eat too much honey…
>
> —PROVERBS 25:16, 27

Earlier in Proverbs, the honeycomb is compared to pleasant words: "sweet to the soul and healing to the bones" (Prov. 16:24). It's proven that unprocessed honey helps our health in multiple ways:

- Aids stomach digestion
- Treats allergies

- Heals ulcers and burns

- Has anticancer properties

- Moisturizes skin

Fit Fact: *The Journal of the American Medical Association* reports, "Applied every 2 to 3 days under a dry dressing, honey promotes healing of ulcers and burns better than any other local application. It can also be applied to other surface wounds, including cuts and abrasions."[5]

So what's Solomon's beef with honey? Well, honey, though a natural substance, is considered refined because it contains large amounts of the simple sugars fructose, sucrose, maltose, and glucose.

A daily overdose of refined sugar can cause the following:

- Excess fat

- Fatty organs and tissues

- Abnormal blood pressure

- Diabetes

- Decrease of body's immunizing power

- Negatively affected brain function and memory

- Depletion of body's B vitamins

- Increased fatigue

- Tooth decay

- Appetite for more sugar!

Fit Fact: The Crusaders who followed Edward I to Palestine died in large numbers from excessive heat and from eating too much honey and fruit.[6]

The biblical principle is simply to use refined carbohydrates in—you guessed it—moderation. Refined carbs include:

- Bread and pasta made with refined flour
- Sweet bakery products, like cookies and cakes
- Refined grains, like white rice
- Most puddings, custards, and other sweets
- Fruit drinks, sodas
- Jelly, jams, and all candy

According to the World Health Organization, no more than 10 percent of calories should come from added sweeteners.[7] For example, if you consume two thousand calories a day, no more than two hundred calories (50 grams) should come from sugar. Read your nutrition labels! A small, 4.2 ounce juice box has nearly 15 grams (4 teaspoons) of sugar. The sugar may be natural, but your body does little to distinguish it from any other kind of sugar.

Don't be deceived by their fancy names. The following is a list of commonly used simple sugars:

- Fructose
- Maltose
- Glucose
- Sucrose (table sugar)
- High-fructose corn syrup
- Sorbitol, mannitol, malitol, xylitol (sugar alcohols)

Fit Fact: Sugars that are added to foods are listed in the foods ingredient list. If one of the terms meaning sugar is listed first, second, or third, sugar is one of the main ingredients. The suffix -ose indicates that the substance is a sugar, but not all sugars end in these letters.

Modern nutritional advice clearly shows us that King Solomon had it right about sugar twenty-nine hundred years ago! What God showed His people way back then is exactly what doctors and scientists are encouraging us to do now:

- Reduce intake of fats

- Limit consumption of meat and refined carbs

- Increase consumption of complex carbs (whole grains, fruits, vegetables)

GOD'S GARDEN SPEAKS FOR ITSELF

My last semester of college I took a nutrition course that taught all about the vital nutrients found in fruits and vegetables as well as which diseases those nutrients help prevent and which bodily functions they facilitate. While studying for my first exam, I tried to cleverly devise an easy way to memorize which food did what. If only I'd known that many of the answers can be found in the food themselves!

If looking up at the night sky isn't enough to make you marvel at our Maker's handiwork, maybe you should try slicing open a tomato. It turns out that a food's mere appearance indicates its importance to our bodies. The following chart illustrates a few examples:

Food	Appearance	Function
Tomato	Red, 4 chambers (like the human heart)	Contains lycopene, an inhibitor of heart disease
Walnut	Looks like a brain, with a left and right side and upper cerebrum and lower cerebellum. Even the wrinkles on the nut resemble the brain's neo-cortex.	Helps develop over three dozen neurotransmitters for brain function.
Celery, bok choy, rhubarb	Look like bones	These vegetables are 23 percent sodium, just like bones. A lack of sodium in the diet forces the body to pull it from the bones, weakening them. These foods replenish the body's skeletal needs.

Food	Appearance	Function
Grapes	Hang in a heart-shaped cluster, and each grape resembles a blood cell.	Contain flavonoids and phytonutrients that decrease risk of heart disease
Kidney beans	A no-brainer: These look like kidneys!	Heal and help maintain kidney function
Sweet potatoes	Look like the pancreas	Balance the glycemic index within diabetics
Eggplant, pears, avocados	Look like a woman's cervix and womb	Balance hormones, help shed unwanted birth weight, prevent cervical cancer. It takes nine months to grow an avocado from blossom to ripened fruit!
Olives	Look like ovaries	Assist the health and function of the ovaries
Oranges, grapefruits, other citrus fruits	Resemble mammary glands of females	Assist breast health and the movement of lymph in and out of the breasts
Carrots	A sliced carrot looks like the human eye	Greatly enhance blood flow to the eyes

Pretty amazing, isn't it? This knowledge gives us even more motivation to eat salads chock-full of garden goodness and enjoy the sweetness of citrus on sweltering summer days. And how fun to know exactly what your pre-workout orange or post-workout sweet potato is doing for your body, besides providing energy and revving up your metabolism.

A COLOR-CODED CORNUCOPIA

Not only can foods' looks give us a clue as to their function, but their colors advertise which vitamins and minerals they feature. I was definitely thankful to know this much while taking my nutrition class.

Color	Nutrients	Functions	Examples
Green	Chlorophyll, calcium, folate, vitamin C, lutein, zeaxanthin	Reduce cancer risks, lower blood pressure and LDL cholesterol levels, normalize digestion time, fight harmful free radicals, boost immune system activity	Green apples, arugula, asparagus, broccoli, lettuce, limes, avocados, zucchini, kiwifruit, green pears, leafy greens, green grapes, okra, peas, artichokes
Red	Lycopene, ellagic acid, quercetin, hesperidin	Lower blood pressure, reduce risk of prostate cancer, reduce tumor growth and LDL cholesterol levels, scavenge free radicals, support joint tissue in arthritis cases	Cherries, red apples, red bell peppers, guavas, red onions, red pears, strawberries, watermelons, tomatoes, red grapes, raspberries, radishes
Orange/ yellow	Beta-carotene, zeaxanthin, lycopene, potassium, flavonoids, vitamin C	Reduce age-related macular degeneration and the risk of prostate cancer, lower blood pressure and LDL cholesterol levels, promote collagen formation and healthy joints, encourage alkaline balance, work with magnesium and calcium to build healthy bones, fight harmful free radicals	Sweet potatoes, pumpkin, oranges, carrots, cantaloupe, papayas, peaches, mangos, pineapples, yellow beets, yellow peppers, yellow summer squash, yellow tomatoes, sweet corn, tangerines, yellow apples, rutabagas

Color	Nutrients	Functions	Examples
Blue/purple	Zeaxanthin, lutein, vitamin C, fiber, flavonoids, quercetin, ellagic acid	Support retinal health, lower LDL cholesterol levels, boost immune system activity, support healthy digestion, improve calcium and other mineral absorption, fight inflammation, reduce tumor growth, limit the activity of cancer cells, act as anticarcinogens in the digestive tract	Blueberries, blackberries, eggplant, purple grapes, pomegranates, prunes, raisins, purple figs
White	Beta-glucans, Epigallocatechin gallate (EGCG), lignans	Provide powerful immune-boosting activity; activate natural killer B and T cells; reduce the risk of colon, breast, and prostate cancers; balance hormone levels; reduce risk of hormone-related cancers	Cauliflowers, dates, jicama, bananas, parsnips, potatoes, Jerusalem artichokes, shallots, white corn, white peaches, white nectarines

So next time you're in doubt in the buffet line, pretend your plate is an artist's palette and load on the colors! After all, God said you were a masterpiece (Ps. 139:14)!

Fit Fact: To save money, buy foods that are in season and grown locally.

4

BEYOND THE PALE

Sickness, Oppression, and Healing

*Dear friend, I pray that you may enjoy good health and that all
may go well with you, even as your soul is getting along well.*
—3 JOHN 2

W E KNOW THAT adhering to God's nutrition plan and maintaining an active lifestyle are the keys to physical—and, in many ways, spiritual—health. But what about when we do get sick, grow weary, or feel depressed? Since Adam and Eve fell, sickness has been a pervasive obstacle that even the healthiest individuals are susceptible to. In this chapter we'll examine the reasons why healthy Christians can fall victim to sicknesses and learn how to overcome them. Be warned; you won't hear this in your health class or read it in your fitness magazine.

WWJD?—WHAT *WOULDN'T* JESUS DO?

Before we address some of the reasons we come down with a cold, the flu, or perhaps something more severe, let's first look at a common misconception many Christians have accepted as truth when it comes to physical ailments.

One of the most prevalent notions in teachings on sickness and healing is that God gives Christians sicknesses and injuries to teach them a lesson or to strengthen their faith. This is simply untrue, and yet it has been disseminated by pastors, teachers, and theologians as a biblical principle. You see, God created us to be perfectly healthy. In fact, the original plan—before Adam and Eve sinned—was that mankind would live forever, just as the angels in heaven do. When sin entered the world, the curse accompanied it as its villainous sidekick, bringing sickness, pain, hurt, and crime into what was once a perfect paradise. This is why there is an innate, God-given aversion to death; man was never intended to perish and still strives for long life.

Fit Fact: According to VisualEconomics.com, the United States spends 19.3 percent of its budget on healthcare expenses.[1]

I've heard people say after recovering from a sickness, "Well, I was pretty miserable, but I know God gave it to me to test my faith!" I've even heard preachers proclaim, "The minute you feel a fever come on you, ask yourself, 'Have I sinned against God?' He may be trying to get your attention!"

Hebrews 1:2 (NKJV) tells us that Jesus is the "express image" of God. The Amplified translation of the Bible says Christ is "the perfect imprint and very image of God's nature." Did Jesus, God incarnate, ever curse a man with leprosy or strike a woman with boils and sores? The answer is absolutely not! Acts 10:38 says Jesus went about "healing all who were oppressed by the devil for God was with Him" (NKJV).

Reading the four Gospels, we see Jesus healing everyone who came to Him believing. Jesus said He did only what He heard His Father say (John 8:28). To believe God is the giver of pestilence and the purveyor of plagues would paint Jesus as an unfaithful follower of God's instructions. Jesus came to give life abundantly, not take it (John 10:10). He would no more make you sick than He would lead you to sin. The cross has redeemed us from sin and sickness both!

Perhaps a fanciful fable can help illustrate God's desire for us to be well.

Tale of three princesses

Once upon a time there lived a great king who ruled a beautiful kingdom and loved his people with all of his heart. The time came when he desired to travel across a great sea to prepare a family reunion filled with the most delicious foods, rarest flowers, and most marvelous music.

Before he left, he asked his son to go to the kingdom's finest stable and purchase the four best horses for him and his sisters to have as a parting gift. The son obeyed and selected four of the most exquisite horses in the kingdom. They were strong and fast, with long, flowing manes and sleek, shining coats.

The son sent the horses chosen for his sisters ahead of him with his servants, and he followed behind on his steed, taking in the beauty of the sunset sinking softly into the hillside. Just miles away from the castle, the son was ambushed by a band of thieves who battered him to death and left him by the roadside.

The other three horses arrived safely to the castle and were put inside a special corral, waiting for the king's daughters to come for them. After the time of grieving for their brother had passed, the daughters excitedly ran to see their new horses—one golden, one snow white, the third black as night. Day after day the daughters fed the horses grains from the cups of their hands, combed and braided their manes, and sat upon them, pretending themselves to be valiant knights and distressed damsels, conquering dragons and saving the innocent.

When the king returned and asked his daughters how they liked the horses, he was grieved to hear that they never once took the horses out of the corral. They never went riding through the kingdom's forests or upon the emerald-green slopes. They never trotted into town to go to the markets, nor used the horses to carry their goods. They never truly enjoyed the horses the way he had intended. They only doted on the majestic creatures and dreamed of what they could be.

The king hung his head and began to weep as he thought of the great price he had paid to provide his children with such wonderful gifts, that of his only son who died delivering them.

> Bless the Lord, O my soul, and forget not all His benefits: who forgives all your iniquities; *who heals all your diseases…*
> —PSALM 103:2, EMPHASIS ADDED

So, why do I get sick sometimes? A very legitimate question. Just because we become saved and redeemed from sin when we accept Jesus as Lord doesn't mean we will never sin again. In the same way, being redeemed from sickness doesn't mean we'll never have to buy a bottle of Tylenol or take Tums again. Generally speaking, many of our problems are due to the fact that we live in a fallen world. For example, if you were living in Eden before the Fall and accidentally cut yourself while slicing a freshly picked apple, it wouldn't hurt, it wouldn't bleed, and the skin would likely mend itself together again before your eyes. Nowadays, if you cut yourself while slicing an apple in your apartment, you'll bleed, maybe fight back tears, and slap on a Band-Aid. Ever since mankind was evicted from Eden, bruises, fractures, sickness, and disease have abounded. There's no getting around the effects of the Fall—unless you get around in a bubble.

The good news is, Christ died for our sins and our diseases. Quoting the Book of Isaiah, Matthew writes, "He took up our infirmities and carried our diseases" (Matt. 8:17). Faith in God's healing atonement through the sacrifice of His Son is what overcomes sickness. The next time you feel your body getting sick, whether it's a stomachache or laryngitis, quote scriptures of healing to the Lord in prayer and believe that you are well. First Peter 2:24 tells us that we were healed by Jesus's stripes. He already paid the price for your healing. All you have to do is believe for its manifestation "on earth as it is in heaven" (Matt. 6:10).

Fit Fact: Research shows crash dieting, anorexia, or nutrient deficiencies increase a person's susceptibility to infections, but overconsumption of calories can also have harmful effects on cell production in the immune system.

AN OPEN DOOR: THE SIN-SICKNESS CONNECTION

Now that we've dismissed the erroneous idea that God gives us sickness, we can delve into the true, spiritual reasons that often lurk behind physical illnesses. As we've seen, sin ushered the existence of sickness into the world. Not much has changed since Adam's day, when he and his wife bit into that forbidden fruit. Just as their sin introduced them to "pains…toil…thorns and thistles," so our sins can open doors to sickness, weakness, and oppression (Gen. 3:16–18).

One of Jesus's many healing miracles involved a man who had been an invalid for thirty-eight years. He, like countless others with various disabilities and diseases, was sitting around the pool of Bethesda waiting for a healing to surface from its waters. Jesus asked the man if he wanted to be made whole. Of course, Jesus is omniscient and knew the man's answer before ever getting a response. Similarly, God knew where Adam was long before He called for him in the garden after Adam sinned. When God asks us a question, He doesn't desire an answer for Himself but acknowledgment and self-examination from us.

Healing comes only to those willing to receive it. Clearly this man wanted to be healed or he wouldn't have been waiting around a crowded public pool day after day with the sun beating down on him. He explained to Jesus that he had no one to help him into the water. Jesus said to him, "Rise, take up thy bed, and walk" (John 5:8, KJV). The man obeyed and was immediately able to walk. But before the newly healed man was able to skip jubilantly away or start training for the Olympics, Jesus admonished him to "sin no more, lest a worse thing come unto thee" (John 5:14). We don't know the details of the man's past, but we can infer from Jesus's cautioning words to him that it was sin that brought about his infirmity.

Faith Fact: The Bible only records a fraction of the miracles Jesus performed. If each one had been recorded, there would not be enough room to hold the books containing them (John 21:25)!

As we discussed in chapter 3, the old-covenant Law was a "school teacher" instructing God's people about His awesome holiness and exposing their exceeding sinfulness (Gal. 3:24; Rom. 7:13). Israel was given strict rules to follow and severe consequences if they broke them, including sicknesses and plagues (Deut. 28:58–60). These rules were given as a standard for right-living for a covenant people, but when Jesus came, He freed us from the Law. As Christians, we're now part of a covenant of grace! (Can I get an "Amen"?) Galatians 3:13 says that "Christ has redeemed us from the curse of the law, having become a curse for us" (NKJV).

When we sin, we cause the hedge of protection that Christ paid for with His blood to be lifted, rendering us vulnerable to the old-covenant effects of disobedience. Addictions, pride, selfishness, anger, bad habits, and everything else that stands in direct opposition to the Word of God negate His promises of protection and blessing in our lives, because we cannot serve two masters (Rom. 6:16). We either live in righteousness through our faith in Jesus Christ or in sin through our rebellion.

PRIDE COMETH BEFORE A FALL: MY PERSONAL SIN

The example of the healed man above is one example of how a person's individual sin can produce sickness. I experienced the ramifications of my own sin when I battled anorexia several years ago.

After my boyfriend of two years broke up with me during my junior year of high school, I felt as if my world was turned topsy-turvy. Instead of drawing near to the Lord and relying on Him to supply my strength and give me comfort, I looked to myself. I turned to working out and food as a means of obtaining control and began hitting the gym harder than before, often twice a day. I counted every calorie that entered my mouth and rarely ate around people or went to restaurants. Before I knew it, my weight had dropped significantly, and my health was declining.

It flattered me to hear friends and peers comment on how thin I had become, even if they did so with worry hanging in their voices. I distinctly remember thinking my best friend was "just jealous" when she confronted me about how dangerously frail I looked one night at a concert. You see, my pride in assuming I could strengthen myself and bring myself joy had supplanted God's grace. And as my efforts increased, so too did the terrible repercussions of pride.

I became obsessed with my appearance. I isolated myself from my friends because I thought they were judging my eating habits and my "disciplined" devotion to working out. I declined invitations to parties and social events if they interfered with my plans to go to the gym. I had given Satan an inroad into my life, and his destructive plan was rapidly unfolding. Depression set in, my hair and nails became dry and brittle, and my skin pale and sallow. I felt heart palpitations, I was consistently cold and unexplainably exhausted, I lost my menstrual cycle, and I even had osteopenia, the precursor to osteoporosis.

It wasn't until I acknowledged, confessed, and repented of my pride that God's healing work could begin restoring me from the inside out. Like the man who had been an invalid, I was both forgiven of my sin and healed of my disease. However, falling back into pride could potentially precipitate similar afflictions. It is only by surrendering to God's strength and having faith in His desire to heal our broken heart and bind up our wounds that we rest in the promises of His provision (Ps. 147:3).

Faith Fact: The Greek word for "save" is *sozo*, which also means "heal."[2]

Keep Your Temple Tidy

Sickness is often a result of our own negligence when it comes to taking care of our bodies. The mistake stems from the notion that we own these temporary tents of flesh and can therefore treat them however we see fit—or unfit, shall we say. We know by now that we are not our own and that God commands that we glorify Him in our bodies (1 Cor. 6:19–20).

Something as seemingly harmless as not getting enough sleep, stressing out over a job application or a college exam, or drinking too many energy drinks is enough to send our health into a downward spiral. In his first letter to Timothy, Paul suggested that he change his diet in order to rid himself of his frequent sicknesses, likely brought on by drinking contaminated water (1 Tim. 5:23). Now, some of you may say, "Yeah, and Paul also told him to use a little wine to help his stomach!" Touché. However, the Bible is consistent in teaching moderation. It doesn't forbid drinking alcoholic beverages, but it does forbid drunkenness (Prov. 23:29–35). Whatever the virtues of using a little wine may be, this verse simply means that substituting wine for water was in Timothy's best interest given the substandard condition of the drinking water in Ephesus.

In Timothy's case, it wasn't prayer that was needed to heal him. The remedy was simply a beverage change. We probably come down with colds and other illnesses due to our own sloppy eating, unnecessary stressing, and inadequate sleeping more often than we'd like to admit. Not caring for our bodies is undeniably a sin that can make us sick, which is exactly what the devil wants us to be.

Faith Fact: A study at the University of Wisconsin found that sustained stress can have a negative impact on immunity. Blood samples taken from stressed-out students taking a final exam showed the ability of natural killer cells to kill cancer cells was reduced.[3]

GOOD-BYE TO GRUDGES

Every Christian worth his or her salt knows forgiveness is a prominent facet of our faith. A well-known parable in Matthew 18:23–35 tells the story of a man whose enormous debt was canceled by a king, and yet he refused to forgive his fellow servant. His forgiveness was then removed, and he was led captive to a life of torment until he could repay the debt. I'm sure you can figure out who's who in the story: God is the king, we are the hypothetical forgiven servant, and the owed sum is our sin. The crux of the parable is not our experience of God's forgiveness but the effects of that forgiveness in our relationships with others.

When we refuse to forgive, we show that we don't truly understand the divine forgiveness imparted to each of us at the cross.

Christ loved us enough to lay down His life so we might be forgiven. Yet how often we fail to incorporate the "as we forgive those who trespass against us" part of the Lord's Prayer into our Christian walks. Holding a grudge against someone for something as minor as forgetting your birthday or as major as spreading a malicious lie about you prevents forgiveness in our own lives, blocks answers to our prayers, and sends an invitation for sickness and oppression to come crash your party.

The Bible is clear about our forgiveness of others:

> And when ye stand praying, forgive, if ye have ought against any: that your Father also which is in heaven may forgive you your trespasses.
>
> —MARK 11:25, KJV

> If we confess our sins, he is faithful and just to forgive us our sins, and to cleanse us from all unrighteousness.
>
> —1 JOHN 1:9, KJV

> But if ye forgive not men their trespasses, neither will your Father forgive your trespasses.
>
> —MATTHEW 6:15, KJV

> Forbearing one another, and forgiving one another, if any man have a quarrel against any: even as Christ forgave you, so also do ye.
>
> —COLOSSIANS 3:13, KJV

> If you forgive anyone his sins, they are forgiven; if you do not forgive them, they are not forgiven.
>
> —JOHN 20:23

Not forgiving others is indeed a sin, like my pride years ago, that opens the door to sickness. We already know that we cannot live in sin and simultaneously expect to receive the blessings our Savior died to give us. Likewise, we cannot enter into prayer with an unforgiving spirit and expect God to be "all ears." Only when we genuinely forgive the one who hurt or offended us and repent of our ill thoughts or actions that have taken root as a result of our own bitterness are our own prayers answered and our sins forgiven.

What if I don't feel like it? Boy, oh boy, have I had to deal with that thought stampeding through my brain like a herd of buffalo when I've tried to justify my way out of forgiving. Turns out, that thought doesn't hold a lot of water. The Word of God does not ask us to feel like it but to make a decision to make like Nike and just do it! Many times I've felt the most forgiving after I obeyed the Lord and showed forgiveness with a loving heart. Remember, our spirit is at war with our flesh (Gal. 5:17). Though our feelings may desire nothing more than to go to the grave with the grudge we've befriended, as new creations no longer bound to sin, the seemingly impossible task of forgiving is made doable and, might I add, enjoyable by the grace of God (Rom. 6:11–14).

Many health experts refer to unforgiveness as a deadly emotion because of its undeniable link to a variety of health issues. Whenever our brain rehearses past wrongs and permits offenses to stew in our psyche, the subsequent release of biochemical stress responses often leads to increased blood pressure, headaches, rapid sweat and heart rates, muscle tension, and a depressed immune system. As unforgiveness is allowed to linger, these natural responses wreak havoc on the body, leading to increased risks of heart disease, cancer, and stroke.

Unforgiveness can also negatively affect our brains. Studies show that even mild resentment and anger tend to lower cognitive function and problem-solving capacity. Mental errors tend to increase, and problems become more difficult to solve. Additionally, unforgiveness can lead to anxiety disorders, depression, and shame.

A study done at Hope College in Michigan asked seventy undergraduate students to remember a time when they were mistreated or harmed by someone. The participants were asked to either practice forgiving or being unforgiving. Their psychophysiological, emotional, and facial responses were all recorded. Those being unforgiving reported feeling sadness, anger, negativity, and a lack of control. Physiologically they showed greater tension in the brow area of the face and higher blood pressure. Their theory was that forgiveness:

> …may free the wounded person from a prison of hurt and vengeful emotion, yielding both emotional and physical benefits, including reduced stress, less negative emotion, fewer cardiovascular problems, and improved immune system performance.…Unforgiving

memories and mental imagery might produce negative facial expressions and increased cardiovascular and sympathetic reactivity, much as other negative and arousing emotions (e.g., fear, anger) do.[4]

Not only is forgiveness great for your spirit, but it's also good for your health. Anyone else feel like forgiving someone, even if it's not necessary?

Faith Fact: In 1988, a Gallup poll found that forgiveness is something 94 percent of Americans aspire to, but 85 percent said they needed "outside help" to effectively forgive. The majority of people said this help comes from meditative prayer.[5]

TIME DOESN'T HEAL ALL WOUNDS; FAITH DOES

Prior to understanding healing and discovering the unavoidable fact that God wants me to be well even more than my own parents do, I always considered sicknesses as "up to God" and "perhaps it's just God's will." I found myself in a trap that many Christians are stuck in today, one that inhibits our service to God, prevents us from receiving the healing Christ paid for, crushes our spirits, and often leads to premature death and unnecessary suffering and frustration.

First Peter 2:24 lets us know there's no sense wondering whether or not God will choose to heal you: "by His wounds you have been healed." Jesus has already provided the healing! He even commanded His disciples—that includes you and me—to continue His work of deliverance, both spiritually and physically, saying:

> Heal the sick, raise the dead, cleanse those who have leprosy, drive out demons. Freely you have received, freely give.
> —MATTHEW 10:8

Faith Fact: Over 20 percent of the gospel is about the healing ministry of Jesus Christ.[6]

Christians today have no problem embracing forgiveness, deliverance, and the gifts of the Spirit as part of the salvation package, so to speak. When we become Christians, we also become new creations (2 Cor. 5:17). If a woman you know who constantly gossiped, stirred up strife, and spread rumors, and had a spirit of jealousy while also battling an illness came to church and received Christ, we would expect her, as a new creation, to be freed from the spirit of jealousy and to repent from her wicked tongue. Why wouldn't we also expect her to be healed from her illness? Each illness associated with the old self has been dealt with on the cross.

Jesus asked rhetorically, "Which is easier: to say, 'Your sins are forgiven,' or to say, 'Get up and walk'?" (Luke 5:23). In practice, it should even be easier to heal sickness than deal with sin. Healing from Jesus required only words, whereas forgiveness required His death.

Most God-fearing Christians know that Jesus is the standard by which we measure our lives. There is absolutely no evidence that Jesus was ever sick. He likely never missed a teaching opportunity at the synagogue because He had a cold. He never declined a request to heal someone because He had food poisoning from undercooked meat. *Yeah, but Jesus is God.* Remember, He was fully God and fully man and therefore was susceptible to sickness just like all of humanity (1 Tim. 2:5). If Jesus was in full health, we should expect the same. Despite the healing provided for us through Jesus, sickness is still pervasive in the church and disregarded as part of life, when in fact it is part of death. The belief that sickness is normal is, in my opinion, one of the most efficient "flaming arrows" Satan shoots into our minds (Eph. 6:16). When we don't defend ourselves against the arrow of deception and then accept the lie as truth, he gains permission to make us sick.

The first step to freeing yourself from an existing sickness is to revoke its permission to be in your body. This is as easy as refusing to remain sick, saying, "I don't want to be this way anymore. This sickness does not belong in my body!"

Canceling permission may not be, at first, sufficient to bring about healing. Remember, we are engaged in a spiritual battle that involves far more than our own willpower versus the maladies of our flesh. Withdrawing permission is crucial in that it takes away the illness's legal right to infect and weaken our bodies. However, if given a chance, the sickness will squat on our property. If the squatting sickness is especially stubborn (say that three times fast), we must destroy its stronghold.

Spiritual strongholds are brought down by the knowledge of God. Many times we find ourselves still entangled with our former incorrect thinking about sickness and fail to recognize the enemy's attack. This is when we should especially go to the Bible and speak God's Word aloud and remind ourselves of God's plan for our health and well-being. For example: "Praise the LORD, O my soul, and forget not all his benefits—who forgives all your sins and heals all your diseases" (Ps. 103:2–3). Nothing is as powerful as God's Word.

Why is speaking Scripture so important? By proclaiming God's Word, we show our belief in His promises and demonstrate our faithful response to His truths. Not only that, but we override the deceptions that have made us sitting ducks for sickness. While in the wilderness for forty days, Jesus was tempted relentlessly by Satan (Luke 4:1–12). Each time Jesus rejected Satan's lies by inserting the truth of God's Word. He stated the scripture most relevant to His situation and claimed it for Himself. Filling our mind and spirit with God's Word brings us into agreement with God, which in turn completely dissipates the lies the devil generates and the world perpetuates.

Even better than recovering from a sickness is preventing one from manifesting in the first place. Speaking words of faith when we first feel an ache in our back, begin coughing in the morning, or start sneezing at work is how we execute the authority God has given us. We can literally speak to our sickness and command it to leave our bodies! Yesterday morning I awoke feeling very congested, and my nose was running to the *Chariots of Fire* theme song. During my devotional time, I commanded the symptoms to leave in Jesus's name and spoke verses of healing. As I write, I can honestly report that I am healthy as can be and worked out yesterday afternoon without ever needing a Kleenex.

FYI, I don't recommend commanding your illness to take a hike while you're in a classroom or business meeting in the midst of your peers and colleagues. The goal is to be freed from sickness, not committed to an asylum! However, a great opportunity to share the gospel arises when friends ask us how we went from under the weather to on top of the world.

THE GREAT PHYSICIAN'S EDIBLE REMEDIES

In Deuteronomy 8:7–9, God informs the Israelites that He is bringing them into a "good land" that's not only blessed with streams, springs, valleys, and hills but also filled with wonderful foods that just so happen to be health and healing powerhouses. Such foods, enumerated in the Scriptures, are only a sampling of the bountiful healing foods God prescribes to us as natural medicine from His divine pharmacy.

Before we move on to the lighter—both literally and figuratively—subject of sweeteners, let's look at some specific foods mentioned in the Bible that have remarkable healing properties.

Food	Verse	Functions	Easy Applications
Raisins	"Strengthen me with raisins, refresh me with apples" (Song of Sol. 2:5).	Relieve constipation, neutralize acids in the blood, help cure anemia and fever, stimulate libido, promote bone and eye health	Toss them in cereals, granola, and even salads. Snack on a handful for a pre-workout boost or during a hike.
Apples	(Song of Sol. 2:5)	Antiviral, lower cholesterol, clean teeth and gums, flush environmental toxins out of the body, reduce risk of heart disease, regulate blood sugar levels	Enjoy one with a tablespoon of natural peanut butter as a snack. No-sugar-added apple juice and unsweetened applesauce, along with a protein shake, make an excellent snack.
Figs	"They gave him water to drink and food to eat—part of a cake of pressed figs and two cakes of raisins. He ate and was revived, for he had not eaten any food or drunk any water for three days and three nights" (1 Sam. 30:11–12).	Lower and control blood pressure, reduce risk of cancer in women, increase bone density, relieve constipation, help cure anemia	Eat dried figs as part of healthy, energizing snack. Add fresh or dried figs to your oatmeal or cereal. Add fresh, quartered figs to your salad.

Food	Verse	Functions	Easy Applications
Pomegranates	"A land with wheat and barley, vines and fig trees, pomegranates, olive oil and honey" (Deut. 8:8).	Help keep arteries clear of clots, reduces risk of heart attack and stroke, lower LDL cholesterol levels, raise HDL ("good") cholesterol levels, prevent cancer, help fight existing cancer cells in the body, reduce inflammation in sore throats	Pure pomegranate juice is full of antioxidants and tastes great too! Drink it plain or mix it with protein powder for a stellar smoothie.
Grapes	"Noah, a man of the soil, proceeded to plant a vineyard" (Gen. 9:20).	Reduce platelet clumping and blood clots, protect against heart disease, used to help cure asthma and migraines, relieve constipation, prevent fatigue, enhance brain health, prevent macular degeneration, protect the body from viruses	Grapes are great served with string cheese as a snack or within a green salad. Enjoy no-sugar-added grape juice as part of a pre-workout energy boost.
Barley	(Deut. 8:8)	Lowers LDL cholesterol levels, may protect against colon cancer, helps maintain larger populations of friendly bacteria, which crowd out disease-causing bacteria	Eat barley flakes in place of oatmeal for breakfast, adding dried fruit and almonds as a sweet bonus. With its firm, chewy texture, it goes great with crunchy veggies in any salad.

Food	Verse	Functions	Easy Applications
Beans and lentils	"Take wheat and barley, beans and lentils, millet and spelt; put them in a storage jar and use them to make bread for yourself" (Ezek. 4:9).	Decrease risk of heart disease, lower cholesterol, prevent normal cells from turning cancerous	Beans: Munch on ½ cup edamame as a snack. Lentils: Combine cooked lentils and chopped sweet peppers to make a delicious cold salad. Season with your favorite herbs and spices.
Millet	(Ezek. 4:9)	Easier to digest than whole grains, millet keeps intestines healthy and the immune system primed, helps cure magnesium deficiencies, promotes good sleep	Serve it warm with milk as an alternative to hot oatmeal. Pop it like popcorn to produce puffed cereal. Use it in any soup, casserole, or side dish instead of rice.
Spelt	(Ezek. 4:9)	Reduces frequency of migraines, helps lower cholesterol, helps reduce risk of type 2 diabetes, helps women avoid gallstones	Buy spelt bread instead of wheat for sandwiches. Trade your cornflakes in for the spelt variety.

Food	Verse	Functions	Easy Applications
Garlic	"We remember the fish we ate in Egypt at no cost—also the cucumbers, melons, leeks, onions and garlic" (Num. 11:5).	Fights infection, the flu, and colds; thins the blood; reduces blood pressure; stimulates the immune system; guards against heart disease	Use it as a flavor enhancer in just about anything, from whole-wheat pasta dishes to roasts and casseroles. Rub it on your face. No joke! This apparently helps reduce pimples and acne problems.
Onions	(Num. 11:5)	Help lower cholesterol and high blood pressure; prevent atherosclerosis (hardening of the arteries); provide relief from colds, coughs, asthma, and bronchitis; provide protection from tumor growth	Combine them with mushrooms, peppers, celery, and tofu for a sizzling stir-fry! Microwave them with peppers to include in a tomato sauce. Use sliced red onion on your turkey sandwich.
Cucumbers	(Num. 11:5)	Improve skin complexion, lower blood pressure	Add diced cucumber to low-fat tuna fish or chicken salad recipes. For a refreshing, easy-to-make gazpacho, purée cucumbers, tomatoes, green peppers, and onions; then add salt and pepper to taste.

Food	Verse	Functions	Easy Applications
Leeks	(Num. 11:5)	Lower LDL cholesterol and raise HDL, reduce risk of prostate and colon cancer, protect against ovarian cancer, help stabilize blood sugar levels	Finely chop them and add them to your salad. Add them to broths and stews for a delicate, sweet flavor. Use them in an omelet or frittata.
Melons	(Num. 11:5)	Help reduce blood pressure; prevent cardiovascular disease, diabetes, and cancer; help alleviate asthma; protect against macular degeneration; promote energy; promote lung health	Combine all types together for one fabulous fruit salad. Puree cantaloupe and peeled peaches in a blender for a delicious cold soup. Add lemon and honey to taste.
Coriander	"The manna was like coriander seed and looked like resin. The people went around gathering it, and then ground it in a hand mill or crushed it in a mortar" (Num. 11:7–8).	Helps reduce inflammation associated with arthritic joints, strengthen the stomach and improve digestion, helps remove phlegm, helps treat digestive disorders such as hepatitis and dysentery, helps alleviate excess menstrual flow	Mince the seeds, leaves, or roots to use as a sweet, citrusy flavoring for your favorite dishes. Use it when making hot sauce, guacamole, and chili sauce.

Food	Verse	Functions	Easy Applications
Olive oil	"Until I come and take you away to a land like your own land, a land of corn and wine, a land of bread and vineyards, a land of olive oil and of honey, that ye may live, and not die" (2 Kings 18:32, kjv).	Helps prevent heart disease and high blood pressure; helps protect against cancer, arthritis, and diabetes; is excellent for the skin	Use extra-virgin olive oil when making salad dressings. Drizzle it over healthy vegetables before serving. Puree extra-virgin olive oil with garlic and your favorite beans using a food processor to make a terrific dip.
Almonds	"Put some of the best products of the land in your bags and take them down to the man as a gift—a little balm and a little honey, some spices and myrrh, some pistachio nuts and almonds" (Gen. 43:11).	Help lower risk of heart disease, lower cholesterol, protect against diabetes, help keep unwanted pounds at bay, help prevent gallstones	Spread some almond butter on whole-wheat toast in the morning. Fill a celery stick with almond butter for a pick-me-up. Sprinkle a small handful over veggies, cereal, and salad. Mix a few into your yogurt along with raisins or other dried fruit.

Food	Verse	Functions	Easy Applications
Honey	"So he reached out the end of the staff that was in his hand and dipped it into the honeycomb. He raised his hand to his mouth, and his eyes brightened" (1 Sam. 14:27).	Kills bacteria, helps relieve asthma symptoms, boosts energy and immunity, helps heal wounds when applied topically	Can be used as a replacement for sugar in most recipes. Drizzle on oatmeal in the morning. Eat it on a piece of whole-wheat toast with a tablespoon of peanut butter.

Fit Fact: Out of 2.4 million deaths in the year 2000, 365,000 were attributed to poor diet and a lack of exercise.[7]

When you pray a healing verse over your sore throat, go for a glass of pomegranate juice and thank God for its divinely endowed ability to heal. Eating curative foods like the ones listed above are part of the healing God has provided.

Just because we can proclaim healing over our bodies when they're afflicted doesn't give us clearance to eat any way we please, forgo working out, and still expect God to come to our rescue when we gain weight or get the flu. God doesn't operate that way. He is a "rewarder of them that diligently seek him," not of those who use Him when it's convenient (Heb. 11:6, KJV). By taking care of ourselves through proper eating and consistent workouts, we show that we are seeking God by glorifying Him with our bodies (1 Cor. 6:20).

Now the sweet stuff!

THE SKINNY ON ARTIFICIAL SWEETENERS

Why Diet Sodas Are the Enemy

My son, eat thou honey, because it is good; and the honeycomb, which is sweet to thy taste.
—PROVERBS 24:13, KJV

T HE POWDERY WHITE wave of artificial sugars has rolled onto American shores, helping crown "low-sugar" and "sugar-free" as successors to the low-carb craze that had dieters deserting the cereal aisle and flocking to bacon-filled freezers ten years ago. I realize it may seem silly to devote an entire chapter to the subject of artificial sweeteners, but I'm just that passionate about helping women steer clear of these calorie-free, sweet-tasting wolves in sugar's clothing.

This fat-fighting fad seems too good to be true. Sodas, salad dressings, syrups, chocolate—all without calories? We all know that if something seems too good to be true, chances are, it is. In this chapter we'll draw back the curtain concealing the truth about these sweet health offenders and their sour effects on our bodies.

NO TIME FOR ASPARTAME

Aspartame is the technical name for the brand names Equal and NutraSweet. It's found in about six thousand products around the world, including carbonated soft drinks, powdered soft drinks, chewing gum, gelatins, confections, puddings, fillings, dessert mixes, frozen desserts, yogurt, tabletop sweeteners, and some pharmaceuticals, such as vitamins and sugar-free cough drops. And it's no wonder aspartame is popular: it's approximately two hundred times sweeter than sugar, tastes like sugar, can enhance fruit flavors, saves calories, and does not contribute to tooth decay. Again, it sounds too good to be true.[1]

Aspartame accounts for over 75 percent of the adverse reactions to food additives reported to the Food and Drug Administration (FDA). According to researchers and physicians who study its adverse effects, the following chronic illnesses can be triggered or worsened by ingesting aspartame:[2]

- Multiple sclerosis
- Brain tumors
- Epilepsy
- Chronic fatigue
- Alzheimer's disease
- Diabetes
- Fibromyalgia
- Birth defects

Composed of aspartic acid, phenylalanine, and methanol, aspartame should be considered a "chemical poison," not a sugar substitute.[3] Let's briefly look at these components individually:

- Aspartic acid: acts as an excitatory neurotransmitter and can lower the seizure threshold, making a seizure more likely; causes cancer as well as rapid growth in cancers
- Phenylalanine: a precursor of the catecholamine neurotransmitters in the brain; elevated levels in the brain have been associated with seizures
- Methanol: a metabolic poison that converts to formaldehyde (embalming fluid) and formic acid (ant sting poison), both of which attack the central nervous system[4]

Fit Fact: Phenylalanine and aspartic acid are amino acids that are normally supplied by the foods we eat; however, they can only be considered natural and harmless when consumed in combination with other amino acids.[5]

According to renowned neurosurgeon, author, and lecturer Dr. Russell Blaylock, "If you want to avoid obesity, metabolic syndrome and cancer, and if you don't want to make your cancer more aggressive, then you need to stay away from these [aspartame and MSG] products."[6]

You read right. This calorie-free substance can actually cause weight gain! Phenylalanine and aspartic acid stimulate the release of insulin. Strong insulin spikes remove all glucose from the bloodstream and store it as fat. This can result in hypoglycemia and sugar cravings, which tempt us to overeat! On top of that, aspartame has been demonstrated to inhibit carbohydrate-induced synthesis of the neurotransmitter serotonin, which signals that the body is satiated. Inhibition of serotonin leads to food cravings, increased carbohydrate consumption, and, ultimately, weight gain.

Fit Fact: A 2005 study conducted at the University of Texas Health Sciences Center reported a 41 percent increased risk of being overweight for every can or bottle of diet soft drink a person consumes each day.[7]

Given the evidence for aspartame's adverse effects, why hasn't it been banned? Thousands of companies are making billions with aspartame-filled products. That being the case, there are unfortunately plenty of proponents who have their own interests and agendas in mind. FDA officials continue to resist proposals from concerned scientists, physicians, and other groups for comprehensive studies regarding the safety of aspartame.

But just because the FDA approves something doesn't mean we have to. God says His "people are destroyed for lack of knowledge" (Hosea 4:6, KJV). Let's be educated about what foods we choose to fuel our bodies with, especially those made in a lab by fallible scientists.

SACCHARIN: KING OF THE TABLETOP SWEETENERS

You probably know it best as the "pink packet" at restaurants. Over one hundred years old and derived from a Chinese plant, saccharin claims to be the most researched sweetener.[8] It's also known as Sweet'N Low, Sweet Twin, and Necta Sweet. Like aspartame, it's found in a variety of products, such as candy, gum, soda, jams, and juice. Though not as frightening as its neighbor in the blue packet, aspartame, saccharine does pose a few risks.

Though the claims are unsubstantiated, many people have reported allergic reactions to saccharin, including headaches, skin eruptions, and diarrhea. In pregnant women, saccharin has the ability to pass through the placenta and remain in the fetal tissue, which is harmful to the child. Further side effects in infants include irritability and muscle dysfunction, which may be due to saccharin's presence in baby formulas. Saccharin is also excreted in breast milk, so mothers should definitely eliminate or restrict their intake.[9]

Like aspartame and other artificial sweeteners, saccharin may promote weight gain. A study conducted by Purdue University in 2008 and published in *Behavioral Neuroscience* found that saccharin actually increased body weight and calorie intake in rats. Granted, our physiology differs greatly from that of rats, but the study was consistent with human clinical studies that documented weight gain associated with the consumption of intensely sweetened foods and beverages.[10]

In 1977 a study was published showing that male rats displayed the growth of cancerous tumors in the bladder when they consumed saccharin. Afterwards, the US Congress allowed saccharin to be sold as long as it was manufactured with a warning label that says it's a potential health hazard; however, the label was removed in 2000 after subsequent studies showed the sweetener was safe for human consumption.[11] Still seems a bit suspicious to me!

WHAT'S NOT OK WITH ACESULFAME-K

This sweetener with the snazzy name is sold under much more pronounceable labels like Sunett and Sweet One. Like aspartame, it's a whopping two hundred times sweeter than sucrose (table sugar) and is used as a flavor enhancer to preserve the sweetness of sweet treats. It's almost always paired with another artificial sweetener in carbonated drinks and is used in nondairy creamers, pudding, and gelatin products, as well as in pharmaceutical products such as liquid and chewable medications.[12]

Due to mediocre tests conducted in the 1970s, requests have been made to retest the additive for carcinogenicity. What was found, even if not absolute, is certainly disturbing. In the animal studies, Acesulfame-K produced breast and lung tumors, several forms of leukemia, and chronic respiratory diseases. According to the Center for Science in the Public Interest (CSPI), large doses of one of Acesulfame-K's breakdown products, acetoacetamide, have been shown to affect the thyroid of several animals, including rabbits and dogs. In 1987, the CSPI urged the FDA not to approve Acesulfame-K as a viable product, but their concerns were ignored.[13]

The jury is still out on whether or not this product is 100 percent safe for consumption, but I wouldn't risk considering this sweet defendant innocent until proven guilty.

Sucralose: The Latest and Greatest of All Sweet Seducers?

Since Splenda, a.k.a. sucralose, hit US stores in 1999, dozens of products have included the sugar wannabe in their diet varieties, providing consumers with a plethora of low-cal treats that don't skimp on taste. From diet junk foods such as sodas, popcorn, and cookies to more "healthy" products like yogurt and protein shakes, this product gets almost as much grocery store attention as celebrity tabloids. And neither are preferable fuels for our brains or bodies.

Many buyers are deceived into thinking Splenda is a natural, perfectly harmless product. The truth is, it isn't natural at all but is rather a chlorocarbon, which is a fancy name for chlorinated sugar. The process of chlorinating sugar involves chemically changing the structure of the sugar molecule itself by substituting three chlorine atoms for three hydroxyl groups in the overall sucrose (sugar) molecule. Chlorine happens to be one angry and highly excitable element. It is used as a biocide in bleach, insecticide, disinfectants, even World War I poison gas. (You might be asking, "Doesn't salt have chlorine too?" Indeed, but table salt is not a chlorocarbon, which means carbon isn't included when molecular chemistry binds sodium and chlorine to form salt.)

Chlorocarbons are neither nutritionally nor metabolically compatible in our bodies. Unable to excrete the ingested poison, the body shunts the substance into the liver, which is the detoxification organ. There the chlorocarbons damage and destroy the liver's metabolic cells. Not very sweet, is it?

In test animals, Splenda produced:[14]

- Swollen livers and kidneys

- Shrunken thymus glands

- Reduced growth rates

- Decreased red blood cell count

- Hyperplasia of the pelvis

- Extension of the pregnancy period

- Aborted pregnancy

- Decreased fetal body weights and placental weights

- Diarrhea

Splenda claims to have been rigorously researched, but not a single long-term human study has been conducted to ascertain any potential health risks. The FDA only relied on a small number of short-term tests before giving it the OK, and each one of those tests was conducted on animals, not humans, by a Splenda manufacturer.[15] Maybe he or she was biased.

Personally, before I researched the charming yellow packet with the whimsical name, I used it often in my oatmeal, tea, and coffee. I soon began to have frequent headaches, lightheadedness, diarrhea, and loss of appetite. A blood test showed I had elevated liver enzymes indicative of chemical toxins present in the body. My dad, a physician, recommended I eliminate Splenda completely, and a few weeks later I was back to normal.

Fit Fact: In 2004 the National Library published 3,001 studies on saccharin, 774 on aspartame, and just 76 on sucralose.[16]

For whatever reason, Splenda and the FDA continue to insist that Splenda is completely safe despite the fact that manufacturers have affixed chlorine, a known poison, onto the natural sucrose molecule three times. The chemical structure of sucralose and the hazards noted in the preapproval research should suggest to us that the risks of this man-made super sweetener far outweigh any calorie-saving benefits.

DOES XYLITOL HAVE IT ALL?

With just 9.6 calories per teaspoon, xylitol weighs in as a naturally nutritious, low-cal sweetener.[17] Found in the fibers of fruits and veggies, corn cobs, and birch tree bark, xylitol is roughly as sweet as sucrose but with substantially fewer calories—two-thirds less, to be exact. Our bodies actually produce 15 grams of xylitol daily from other food sources.

Xylitol was known to the world of organic chemistry as early as 1891 when it was first manufactured by German chemist Emil Fischer, but it wasn't until World War II that it was rediscovered and made famous by the Finns after a sugar shortage sent them searching for a sweet alternative. It was also during this time that scientists discovered the sweetener's insulin-independent nature, which makes it safe for diabetics.

Though xylitol and sugar look and taste alike, they couldn't be more different. Whereas sugar wreaks havoc on the body by suppressing the immune system, contributing to weight gain, and depleting the bones, to name a few, xylitol does the following:[18]

- Builds immunity

- Has anti-aging benefits

- Protects against chronic degenerative diseases

- Prevents growth of bacteria

Xylitol has been hailed by dentists as "tooth-friendly" due to its ability to help prevent dental caries and cavities as well as ward off plaque. This fact is legitimized by the FDA, which allows xylitol products to advertise their hygienic properties. Xylitol is so popular in countries such as Japan, South Korea, and Sweden that virtually all of their chewing gums contain it.

Fit Fact: According to the American Dental Association, 75 percent of American adults over thirty-five suffer from some form of periodontal disease, such as gingivitis.[19]

Xylitol is great for cooking, perks up your coffee and oatmeal without an unpleasant aftertaste, and has no adverse effects. However, consuming it in large quantities may cause diarrhea or slight cramping. I personally have made the switch from chewing gum with artificial sweeteners to those with xylitol, not only to avoid the harmfulness of the fake stuff but also to help keep my teeth and gums happy. A sugar substitute that tastes like sugar, has few calories, is completely natural, and dentist-approved? Now that's something to smile about!

STEVIA: A NATURAL, NO-CAL TASTE OF THE SWEET LIFE?

A lesser known alternative to table sugar, stevia, is slowly but surely giving sweeteners synthesized in a lab a run for their makers' money. The species *Stevia rebaudiana*, commonly known as "sweet leaf," or simply stevia, has been used for centuries by the Guarani Indians of Paraguay for medicinal and flavoring purposes.[20] The substance occurs naturally as a shrub in tropical and subtropical regions and is completely natural. The leaves of this small green plant have a refreshing taste that can be up to three hundred times sweeter than sugar.

Unlike its artificial counterparts, stevia has been shown to contain several health benefits:

- Aids in weight loss because it contains no calories
- Doesn't adversely affect blood glucose levels and may be freely taken by diabetics
- Tends to lower elevated blood pressure while not affecting people with normal blood pressure
- Inhibits the growth and reproduction of oral bacteria and other infectious organisms
- Improves digestion and soothes upset stomachs

The FDA's position on stevia is ambiguous, because they claim there is simply not enough proof to draw a solid conclusion on its safety, despite dozens of studies that have found the substance to be totally nontoxic. Citing a preliminary study in 1991, the FDA issued an alert that effectively prohibited stevia from being imported into this country. Ironically, this was also the year in which a follow-up study found flaws in the preceding one and questioned its methods and results. The FDA revised its alert in 1995 and allowed stevia and stevia extracts to be imported not as a sweetener but as a supplement.[21] The revision suspiciously sounds like an FDA-mediated compromise between artificial sweetener and sugar lobbyists and the natural food industry. Whatever the reason for stevia's labeling limitations, I'm simply glad it's allowed to be sold.

Fit Fact: According to the president of the Herb Research Foundation, Rob McCaleb, stevia is "safe and intensely sweet, which could make it a popular noncaloric sweetener."[22]

Stevia is the only sugar alternative that is full of pros and absolutely zero cons. Even better, it's so natural that Adam could have sprinkled it on Eve's morning cup of joe. Find it in your local health food store and kiss the toxic time bombs good-bye!

6

CIRCUIT TRAINING
The Great Time Saver

The glory of young men is their strength, gray hair the splendor of old.
—PROVERBS 20:29

W ELL, LADIES, THE time has come for us to get off our comfy couches and into those cute gym clothes. In this chapter we are going to embark upon a fresh, fun, efficient way to work out that requires little or no equipment, half the time of an average workout, and can be done just about anywhere. Don't forget to make sure that you are cleared to exercise by your physician.

Circuit training is an incredible exercise plan that hits all portions of the body as it improves stamina, builds strength, and incinerates calories. A circuit is simply a group of exercises. Each exercise endures for a given interval of time, anywhere from fifteen seconds to two minutes or for a given number of repetitions. After you complete a circuit, you immediately hop to the next one—literally, if you want. The time between each exercise is substantially shorter than that of your average workout routine because the goal is to keep your heart pulsing at a high rate, which equals a calorie-blasting boost in your metabolism.

An additional beauty of circuit training is that its possibilities are utterly endless. From the equipment utilized to the time of the intervals, it is impossible to grow bored or, worse yet, stop seeing and feeling results in your strength, energy, and muscle tone. Whether your goal is to trim down or firm up, circuit training is your ticket to Fit City!

Fit Fact: The renowned Cooper Institute says circuit training is "the most scientifically proven exercise system. It's time efficient and incorporates strength, flexibility and cardio in the same workout."[1]

HOME IS WHERE THE HEALTH IS—CIRCUIT TRAINING IN YOUR LIVING ROOM

Whether you work from a home office, are cutting back due to the present downward economy, or are a stay-at-home-mom, there's no better place to get your workout in than where you hang your hat and rack your dumbbells. By circuit training at home, you can now save both money and time without forgoing the quality of a state-of-the-art health club. In this section we'll see you can never underestimate the power of simplicity.

In the following pages I'm going to give you four incredible routines that will leave you wondering why you haven't experienced the wonders of circuit training sooner. In the first routine, the only piece of equipment you'll need is your body as we focus on stamina and sculpt muscles! In the second, we'll incorporate resistance bands, dumbbells, and an exercise ball to add fat-burning, muscle-building intensity. The third and fourth routines will focus solely on your upper and lower body, respectively.

Oh, and grab a watch that has a second hand!

ROUTINE A

Perform Routine A two days a week and Routine B one day a week for three to four weeks, then reverse the sequence for another three to four weeks so Routine B is done twice and A once. For example:

Weeks 1–4	Routine	Weeks 5–8	Routine
Monday	A	Monday	B
Wednesday	B	Wednesday	A
Friday	A	Friday	B

After two months, you'll be ready to graduate to Routines C and D, which will focus on your upper and lower body individually.

Equipment needed

- Body
- Wall
- Sturdy chair

Do the exercises below for forty-five seconds each in the order listed, moving from one exercise to the next without resting. Complete the circuit three times before moving on to the next, and only rest if you need to.

Note: With any exercise routine, it's important to warm up for at least five minutes so your muscles are warmed and your heart rate reaches a workable rate for beginning exercise. Do a few minutes of jumping jacks, jogging or biking around the block, or running in place.

Circuit 1

Body squat
Position your feet slightly wider than hip-width apart.

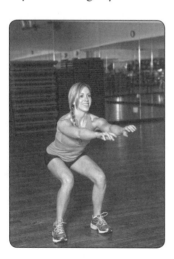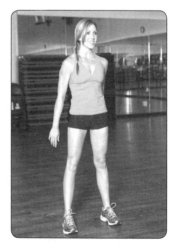

Hold your hands out in front of you at shoulder height for balance.
Slowly bend your knees and lower yourself as far as you can without lifting your heels off the floor.

Pause briefly at the bottom before pushing your weight back up to starting position.

Triceps dips

Sit in a stable chair. Place you hands on the chair slightly wider than hip-width apart.

Walk your feet out in front of you so that your lower back is grazing the edge of the chair. Knees remain at a 90-degree angle.

Lower your body by bending at the elbow. Elbows should not point away from your body as you lower.

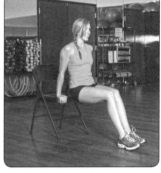

Push heels into the floor as you straighten your arms.

Crunches

Find a comfortable surface (not your bed!), and lie down on your back. Bend your knees, placing your hands behind your head or across your chest.

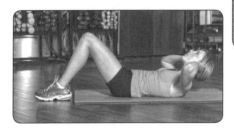

Pull your navel in toward your spine, and press your lower back into the floor.

Slowly squeeze your abs as you bring your shoulder blades 1 to 2 inches off the floor.

Exhale as you come up, keeping your neck straight and chin up.

Slowly lower back down, but maintain a contraction.

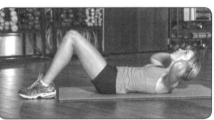

Modified push-ups

Get on your hands and knees. Spread your hands so that they are slightly wider than the width of your shoulders.

Make sure your arms are perpendicular to the floor; move your shoulders to adjust.

Bend your arms as your body slowly lowers to the floor. Make sure your entire body is straight by keeping your navel pulled in toward your spine.

Concentrate on your chest muscles as you push your body back up to starting position.

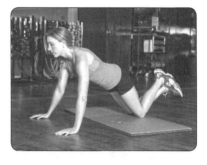

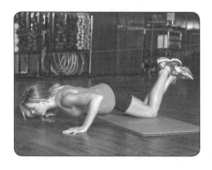

Star jumps

With feet close together, bend your knees to a 90-degree angle.

Bend at the waist so that your torso rests on your thighs. Arms are relaxed over your legs so that hands rest above your feet.

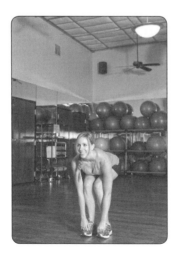
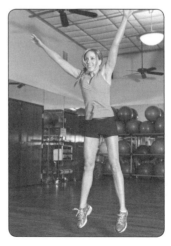

Explode up, taking your hands and feet up and out to create the shape of a star. Focus on squeezing your upper back muscles.

Keep your abs pulled in as you land, and focus on landing softly before exploding up again.

Circuit 2

Knee-to-elbow

Assume a regular push-up position on the floor with hands slightly wider than shoulder width.

Contracting your abs, lift your right leg off the floor, bend your right knee, and bring the knee toward your right elbow as you engage the right side of your oblique muscles. Maintain a flat back throughout the movement.

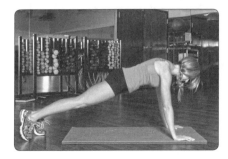 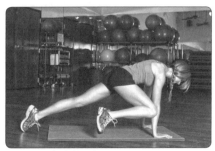

Slowly return to starting position with your right toes on the floor.

Burpees

Get in a squat position with your feet close together and hands on the floor in front of you. With hands on the floor, kick your feet back so that you are in a push-up position.

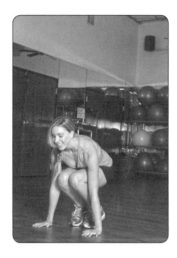 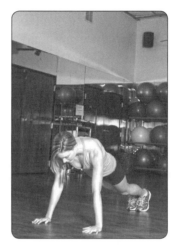

Immediately return your feet to the squat position. Jump up as high as you can from the squat position. Repeat as fluidly as possible.

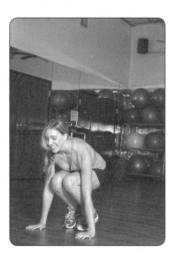 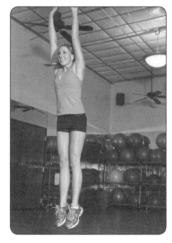

Superman

Lie face down on a soft surface with arms extended overhead. Keep your neck in a neutral position.

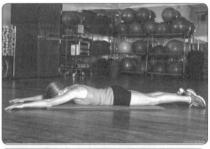

Keeping your arms and legs straight (not locked) and torso stationary, lift your arms and legs toward the ceiling as if to form a *U* with your body.

Hold arms and legs a few inches off the floor for 2 to 5 seconds, and gently lower them.

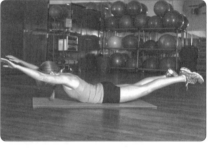

Close-arm wall push-ups

Face a wall, standing an arm's length away. Feet are slightly apart and legs are straight, with your weight in your toes.

Place your hands on the wall with your index fingers and thumbs forming a triangle. Keep your arms in line with your shoulders.

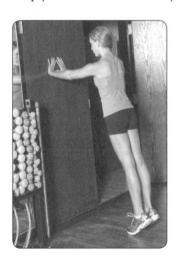
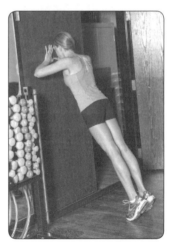

Bend elbows about 90 degrees, and lower your body toward the wall without touching it.

Straighten your arms and return to the starting position.

Note: To make this more difficult, move your feet farther away from the wall.

Circuit 3

Stationary lunges

Stand with your feet as wide as you comfortably can with your right foot in front of your left, left heel lifted, and all toes pointing forward.

Slowly bend your right knee and lower your left knee until it nearly touches the floor. Keep your right knee in line with your right ankle, and do not let your knee move beyond the line of your toes. Your leg should form a 90-degree angle.

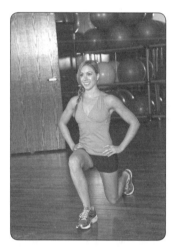 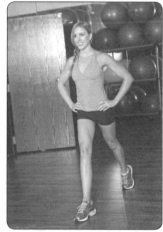

Move straight back up to standing position.

Return your right foot to the center, bring left foot in front, right foot to the back, and repeat.

Continue to alternate right and left for the duration of the 45-second set.

Bicycle crunches

Lie face-up on the floor and lace your fingers behind your head. Keep your elbows back.

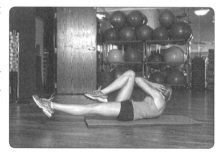

Bring your knees in toward your chest and lift shoulder blades off the ground without pulling on your neck.

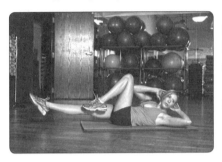

Straighten the left leg out while simultaneously twisting your upper body to the right, bringing the left elbow toward the right knee.

Switch sides, bringing your right elbow toward the left knee.

Double punch

Stand with your feet hip-width apart, knees bent, and with your torso almost parallel to the floor.

"Pin" your elbows to your sides, hands close to your chest.

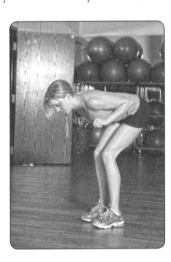 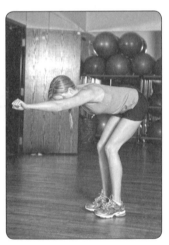

Extend your left arm forward with a closed fist (palm down) as you extend your right arm backward with a closed fist (palm up). Squeeze the muscles of your triceps and shoulder blades.

Bring your arms back to the center and switch sides.

Bridge

Lie on your back with your feet hip-distance apart and your knees bent. Allow your arms to rest at your sides.

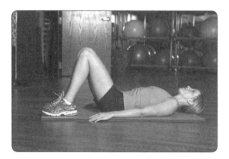 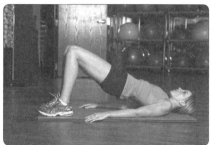

Contract your abs and pull your hips up by tightening your glutes until your body forms a diagonal from knees to chest.

Drop your hips slowly back to the ground, keeping your abs pulled in.

Note: Cooling down is just as important as warming up. It assists in the body's recovery and brings you back to a pre-workout state. It helps your breathing and heart rate return to normal and also prevents dizziness. Gentle aerobic activity like walking for five minutes is an effective cool-down period.

Stretch Descriptions

Note: All stretching photos are located at the end of the workout section.

Hips/glutes
Cross your left foot over right knee.
Grasp your hands behind your right thigh and gently pull your thigh toward you, keeping the body relaxed.
Hold for at least fifteen seconds before switching sides.

Inner thigh
Sit on the floor with your feet pressed together.
Keep your abs pulled in as you lean forward.
Keep leaning until you feel a nice stretch in your inner thighs.

Hamstring
Lie on the floor with your knees bent.
Straighten one leg up toward the ceiling, and slowly pull it toward you, clasping your hands behind the thigh, calf, or ankle—whichever is most comfy.
Keep your knee slightly bent. Hold this position for at least fifteen seconds before switching sides.

Chest and shoulders
Standing, interlock your fingers behind your back, arms straight.
Keeping your hands together, lift them as high as you comfortably can.
Hold for at least fifteen seconds.

Upper back
Clasp your hands together in front of your chest, arms straight.
Round your back toward the floor, pressing your arms away from your body
to feel a stretch in your upper back.
Hold for at least fifteen seconds.

Triceps
Standing, bend your right elbow behind your head and use your left hand
to gently pull the right elbow in further until you feel a stretch in the back of
your arm (triceps).
Hold for at least fifteen seconds before switching sides.

Spine twist
Lie on the floor and place your right foot on your left knee.
Using your left hand, gently pull your right knee toward the floor, twisting
your spine, keeping your hips and shoulders on the floor and your left arm
straight out.
Hold for at least fifteen seconds before switching sides.

Circuit 1

Exercise	Muscle Groups	Time
Body squat	Glutes, thighs	45 seconds
Triceps dips	Triceps, chest	45 seconds
Crunches	Rectus abdominis (long muscle of the abdomen, a.k.a., the "six pack" muscle)	45 seconds
Modified push-ups	Chest, triceps, abs	45 seconds
Star jumps	Whole body	45 seconds

Circuit 2

Exercise	Muscle Groups	Time
Knee-to-elbow	Obliques	45 seconds
Burpees	Whole body	45 seconds
Superman	Lower back	45 seconds
Close-arm wall push-ups	Triceps, chest	45 seconds

Circuit 3

Exercise	Muscle Groups	Time
Stationary lunges	Thighs, glutes	45 seconds
Bicycle crunches	Rectus abdominis, obliques	45 seconds
Double punch	Shoulders, upper back	45 seconds
Bridge	Thighs, glutes	45 seconds

Note: Remember to cool down before stretching.

Stretch	Time
Hips/glutes	15–30 seconds on each leg
Inner thigh	15–30 seconds
Hamstring	15–30 seconds on each leg
Chest and shoulders	15–30 seconds
Upper back	15–30 seconds
Triceps	15–30 seconds on each arm
Spine twist	15–30 seconds on each side

Stretching

After you cool down, take a few minutes to stretch the worked muscles. Doing so improves circulation, increases flexibility, helps maximize the range of motion in your joints, and reduces soreness and stress! Each stretch should be held between fifteen and thirty seconds and should feel good. If it becomes painful, ease up a bit, breathe deep, and go slower.

Routine B

In this routine, we'll be incorporating equipment that you may or may not be familiar with. If you don't own the following already, I strongly encourage you to consider making them a part of your home gym:

- Dumbbells

- Resistance bands

- Exercise ball

Dumbbells

Of course, we all know what dumbbells are, but why have them in our homes? Well, dumbbells are quite simply a workout staple. They are the meat to a treadmill's potatoes. They're the Sonny to the bicycle's Cher. And they've withstood the test of time.

The word *dumbbell* originated in the sixteenth century when novice church bell ringers found they'd better gain some brawn to do their job adequately. To develop their arm strength, the ringers connected a rope to a metal weight and swung it against imaginary bells, which produced no sound; hence, it was a dumb bell. In the eighteenth century, dumbbells became the first pieces of home gym equipment. One hundred years later the short bar we know today replaced the rope, and rounded weights were attached at either end.[2]

Dumbbells ensure a balanced workout because they effectively train every muscle group. They offer an increased range of motion, guarantee a challenge so you don't plateau, are completely portable, and most importantly, they're affordable.

What you need:

- If you're brand new to weight training, I suggest purchasing a pair of 5-, 8-, and 10-pound dumbbells. When the 10 pounders become too light, move up to 12, 15, and even 20 pounds.

- If you've been lifting weights for a while, I recommend buying weights in 5-pound increments, from 5 pounds up to 30.

Resistance bands

I was introduced to resistance bands a couple of years ago by a trainer friend of mine, and boy, am I glad I met them! They are ultra-versatile and even more portable than dumbbells, leaving me with no excuses *not* to work out, even when I travel.

With free weights, such as dumbbells, gravity dictates where the weight is coming from, so you feel more resistance as you contract your muscles—e.g., lifting dumbbells up when you do bicep curls—than when you release then tension. However, with bands, the tension is constant, adding a muscle-sculpting challenge.

Bands may seem baffling at first. I mean, they're not exactly a straightforward machine with easy-to-follow directions on them. On the contrary, they're a simple, flimsy-looking apparatus that more resemble a jump rope than a hard-core workout apparatus. They will take some getting used to, but I promise, after you use them and learn the exercises I'm going to teach you, you'll be a believer in bands!

Note: There are different kinds of resistance bands out there to choose from, but let's keep it simple. Choose the basic bands that are long, elastic tubes with padded handles at either end.

What you need:

- Buy a variety of bands. Most are color-coded according to tension level. I recommend having at least a light, medium, and heavy band, because different muscle groups will require different tensions.

- Look for those with padded handles at almost any store, including discount stores.

Exercise ball

Also known as a Swiss ball, exercise balls were originally used by physical therapists and chiropractors in Switzerland for rehabilitation purposes. Through seminars and classes, the bright, bouncy ball was introduced to the United States in the 1980s and made a splash. It was then that athletic trainers, personal trainers, and coaches began using it for their clients and players.

Today, exercise balls are one of the most popular workout tools. They improve balance, flexibility, and add strength to the abs and lower back. It can also be used as a bench in weight-bearing exercises to target hard-to-reach stabilizer muscles, such as the deep abdominal muscles. Exercise balls are also excellent for stretching exercises and can help alleviate back pain and prevent pain from occurring.

What you need:

- Before purchasing your ball, make sure you get the size that best fits you. This depends on your height. If you are:

   4'11"–5'3", you should get a 55 cm ball.

   5'4"–5'10", you should get a 65 cm ball.

   5'11" or taller, you should get a 75 cm ball.

- Also, I recommend buying a ball that is anti-burst or burst resistant.

Optional: floor mat

I suggest purchasing a floor mat if you have hardwood floors or don't want to risk getting carpet burn.

Equipment needed

- Light and medium resistance bands
- A light- and medium-weight pair of dumbbells
- An exercise ball

Do the exercises below for forty-five seconds each in the order listed, moving from one exercise to the next without resting. Complete the circuit three times before moving on to the next, and only rest if you need to.

Note: Remember to warm up, as you did in Routine A.

Circuit 1

Lateral lunge with shoulder press
Stand with the dumbbells hovering at your shoulders.

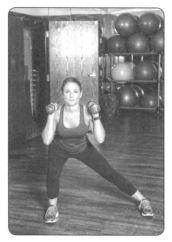 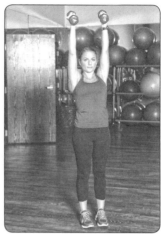

Step to the right and lower your hips to the floor by squatting back and down with the right leg. Keep your left leg straight.

Return to your starting position by pushing up through the right heel and then pressing dumbbells overhead.

Alternate legs and repeat this for the duration of the set.

Dumbbell chest flies

Holding dumbbells, sit on the exercise ball.

Gently roll down until you can relax your head on the ball.

Position your ankles directly under your knees, and lift your hips so they are parallel with the floor; this engages your hamstrings and glutes.

Push the dumbbells over your chest so your palms face each other.

Slowly bring your arms apart as you open your chest.

Keep lowering your arms until they are even with the midline of your chest. Make sure your elbows are not locked and that your knuckles remain facing inward.

Slowly bring the dumbbells up to the starting position over your chest.

Bent-over row
Stand with your knees bent and your torso at a 60-degree angle.

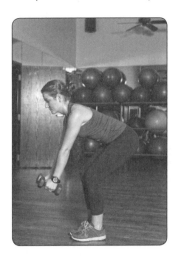 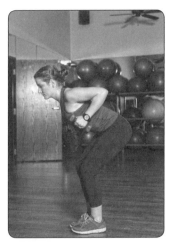

With the weights fully extended in your hands, bring them straight up to your chest, contracting your shoulder blades fully.

Slowly return them to the starting position.

Triceps extension
Hold one handle of the resistance band in each hand.

Position one foot in front of you and the other behind, stepping on the band. Your feet should be about three feet apart.

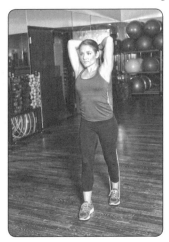 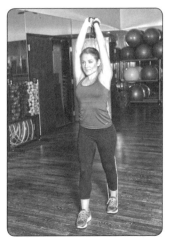

Lift your arms so that the handles are behind your head and your elbows are bent slightly to the sides.

Slowly extend your arms straight over-head and pause, squeezing your triceps before returning to the starting position.

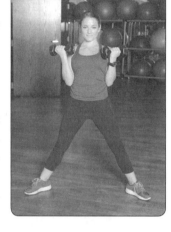

Circuit 2

Plié squat with dumbbell curl

Stand with your feet shoulder-width apart and your toes pointed out, holding a dumbbell in each hand with your arms extended, palms up.

Bend your knees 90 degrees, squatting as you curl the weights toward your shoulders.

Return to the starting position.

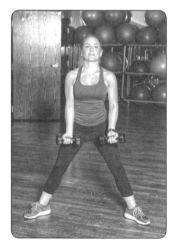
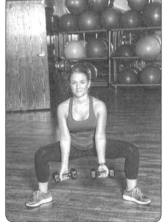

Dumbbell chest press

Holding dumbbells, sit on the exercise ball.

Gently roll down until your upper back rests on the ball, and position the

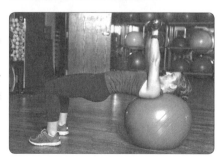

dumbbells so they are even with the midline of your chest, palms facing out in front of you.

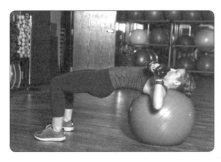

Press the dumbbells up toward the ceiling without locking your elbows. Squeeze your chest muscles.

Slowly lower your arms to the starting position.

Reverse flies

Balance your core on the ball, facing down. Your legs are straight, and your toes are on the floor.

Hold the dumbbells to the left and right side of the ball underneath your shoulders with arms extended.

Raise your arms to your sides, bringing the dumbbells level with your shoulders. Keep your arms as straight as possible without locking your elbows. Keep your neck neutral, in line with the spine.

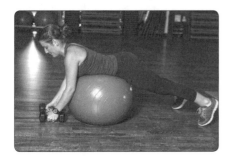
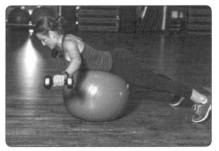

Slowly lower the dumbbells to your starting position.

Ball pass

Lie faceup on a soft surface with your legs straight up (bend them if necessary).

Hold the ball straight over your upper body.

Place the ball between your feet, squeezing them to keep the ball in place.

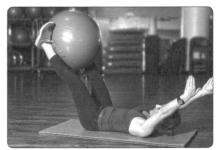

Lower your arms and legs toward the floor, arms reaching backward.

Lift your legs and raise your arms to continue passing the ball from your feet to your hands.

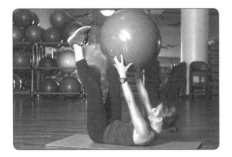 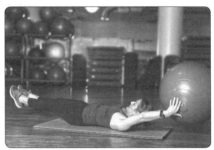

Be careful not to arch your back. To make this easier, bend your knees or decrease your range of motion.

Circuit 3

Alternating lunges with oblique twist

Stand upright while holding the dumbbell out in front of you just below chest level. Don't lock your elbows.

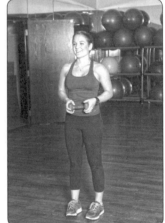

Step forward with your right leg, and lower your body to 90 degrees at both knees. Remember, don't let your knee go past the line of your toes.

As you step forward, rotate your torso to the right side with the dumbbell, keeping your arms straight out in front of you.

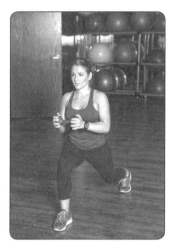 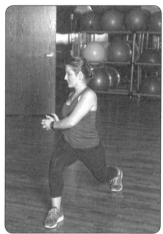

Push back to a standing position with your right leg, and bring your arms back to the center of your body.

Repeat on the left side and continue to switch for the duration of the set.

Decline push-ups

Kneel behind the ball, then place your midsection on it. Roll forward until your hands reach the floor.

Walk your hands out until the ball is underneath your knees. Your hands should be shoulder-width apart. Your body should be as straight as possible.

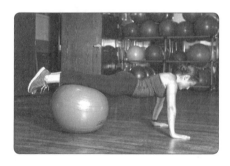 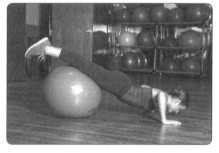

Lower your upper body, bending elbows to 90 degrees.

Straighten your arms as you return to the starting position.

Note: This exercise can be made tougher by moving your feet closer to the ball. Conversely, you can make it easier by bringing your hips closer to the ball.

Biceps curl

Holding either end of the resistance band, stand in the center of the band with your feet and hands shoulder-width apart, palms facing up.

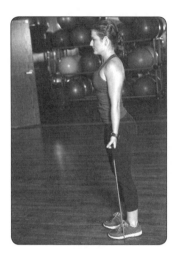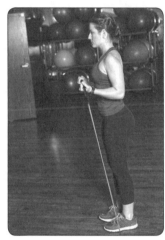

Your elbows are in a fixed position close to your sides.

With control, lift the weight directly up while focusing on your biceps.

Stop when the weight is 90 degrees from your shoulder joints, and reverse the motion down slowly.

Lower your arms, stopping just before your elbows are straight, and reverse the motion back up.

Exercise ball crunch

Sit on the ball and walk your body forward until your hips are just off the ball and your back is on the ball.

Keep your feet about shoulder-width apart, and place hands behind your head. Keep your elbows facing out.

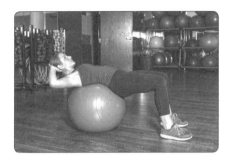 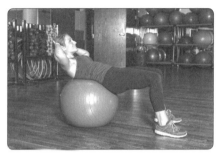

While keeping your hips and lower body still, crunch forward and lift your shoulder blades off the ball.

Hold for one second at the top, and then slowly curl down to starting position.

Stretching descriptions

Quadriceps stretch

Grab a stationary object, like a chair, for balance with one hand.

Use the opposite hand to grasp your leg around the ankle, lifting it toward the buttocks.

Keep your back straight.

Hold and switch legs.

One-arm chest stretch

Stand against the wall. While facing the wall, raise your right hand out to your side at chest height, palm against the wall.

Turn your body toward the left, away from the wall and your extended arm, until you feel a stretch.

Hold and switch sides.

Hamstring stretch

Sit on the floor and extend one leg out straight.

Bend the other leg at the knee and position the sole of that foot against your opposite inner thigh.

Extend your arms and reach forward over the straight leg by bending at the waist as far as possible.

Hold and switch legs.

Back extension

Lie on your stomach.

Prop yourself up on your elbows, extending your back.

Begin straightening your elbows until you feel a gentle stretch.

Upper back

Clasp your hands together in front of your chest, arms straight.

Round your back toward the floor, pressing your arms away from your body to feel a stretch in your upper back.

Hold for at least fifteen seconds.

Triceps

Standing, bend your right elbow behind your head and use your left hand to gently pull the right elbow in further until you feel a stretch in the back of your arm (triceps).

Hold for at least fifteen seconds before switching sides.

Spine twist

Lie on the floor and place your right foot on your left knee.

Using your left hand, gently pull your right knee toward the floor, twisting your spine, keeping your hips and shoulders on the floor and your right arm straight out.

Hold for at least fifteen seconds before switching sides.

Circuit 1

Exercise	Equipment Needed	Muscle Groups	Time
Lateral lunge with shoulder press	Pair of light-weight dumbbells	Glutes, thighs, shoulders	45 seconds
Chest flies	Pair of dumbbells, exercise ball	Chest, core, hamstrings, glutes	45 seconds
Bent-over row	Pair of dumbbells	Upper back, biceps	45 seconds
Triceps extension	Light resistance band	Triceps	45 seconds

Circuit 2

Exercise	Equipment Needed	Muscle Groups	Time
Plié squat with biceps curl	Pair of medium-weight dumbbells	Glutes, inner and outer thighs, biceps	45 seconds
Dumbbell chest press	Pair of medium-weight dumbbells, exercise ball	Chest, core, hamstrings	45 seconds
Reverse flies	Light-weight dumbbells, exercise ball	Upper and lower back, hamstrings	45 seconds
Ball pass	Exercise ball	Lower abdominals	45 seconds

Circuit 3

Exercise	Equipment Needed	Muscle Groups	Time
Alternating lunges with oblique twist	One heavy dumbbell	Thighs, glutes, hamstrings, obliques	45 seconds
Decline push-ups	Exercise ball	Chest, triceps, abs	45 seconds
Biceps curls	Medium-weight resistance band	Biceps	45 seconds
Exercise ball crunch	Exercise ball	Rectus abdominis	45 seconds

Note: Remember to cool down, as you did in Routine A.

Stretch	Time
Quad stretch	15–30 seconds on each leg
One-arm chest stretch	15–30 seconds
Hamstring stretch	15–30 seconds on each leg
Back extension	15–30 seconds
Upper back	15–30 seconds
Triceps	15–30 seconds on each arm
Spine twist	15–30 seconds on each side

ROUTINE C (UPPER BODY)

Give your legs a break! In this circuit routine we'll be letting our arms, shoulders, and abs do all the work. Working upper body on one day and lower on another is technically called a split. This approach allows us to focus our attention on individual muscles and gives those muscles more time to reenergize and recover. Making a change from total-body routines to those that are split-based prevents the body from being overtrained and keeps us away from that dreaded plateau.

Perform Routine C two days a week and Routine D one day a week for three to four weeks. Then reverse the sequence for another three to four weeks so Routine D is done twice and C once. For example:

Weeks 1–4	Routine	Weeks 5–8	Routine
Monday	C	Monday	D
Wednesday	D	Wednesday	C
Friday	C	Friday	D

After two months, return to the total-body format presented in Routines A and B.

Do the exercises below in the order listed, moving from one exercise to the next without resting. These exercises will not be timed, but you should complete the given number of repetitions as you concentrate on proper form and controlled breathing, exhaling during exertion. Complete the circuit three times before moving on to the next. Rest fifteen to thirty seconds between circuits.

Note: Remember to warm up, as you did with the total-body routines.

Equipment needed

- Light and medium resistance bands
- A light, medium, and heavy pair of dumbbells
- Exercise ball
- A chair

Circuit 1

Military press

Holding the dumbbells, sit in the middle of the exercise ball. Sit up straight, and keep your abdomen tucked in. Knees are 90 degrees to the floor.

Raise the dumbbells so they are even with your shoulders, palms facing out.

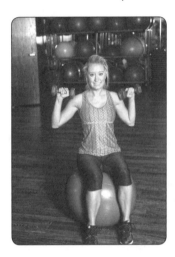 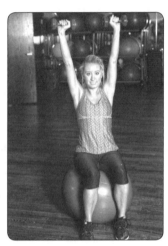

Raise the weight overhead without locking your elbows.

Lower the weight to the starting position.

Dumbbell pull-over

Holding the dumbbell, sit on the exercise ball. Gently roll yourself down so that your shoulders, neck, and upper back rest comfortably on the ball. Make sure your feet are planted firmly on the ground. Contract your hamstrings and glutes to hold yourself in a bridge position.

Position the dumbbell over your chest, placing your hands around the end of the dumbbell farthest from your chest.

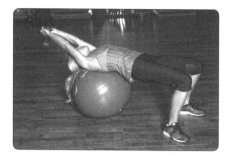 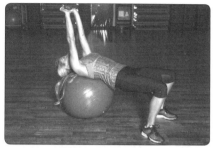

As you inhale, bring the dumbbell behind your head as you slightly bend your elbows and squeeze your chest.

Exhale as you bring your arms back to the starting position.

Incline chest press

Grab the dumbbells. Lie on the ball so that your head, neck, and back are comfortably positioned on the ball. Place your feet firmly on the floor with your knees bent and your rear a few inches from the floor.

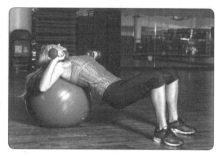

Position dumbbells so they are even with the midline of your chest, palms facing out.

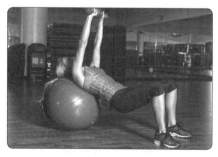

Extend the weights straight up, directly above your collarbone. Do not lock your elbows.

Lower them to the starting position.

Single arm lat pull-down

Stand with your feet shoulder-width apart. Grasp either handle of the band and raise your arms over your head so they are slightly wider than shoulder-width apart.

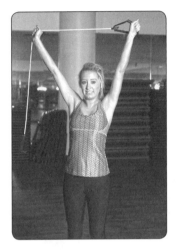 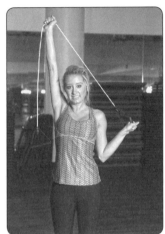

Choose one arm to remain in place as an anchor. Pull the other arm down and to the side until the upper arm is below parallel to the floor.

Slowly return to the starting position.

Circuit 2

Dumbbell push-ups with alternating row

Place the dumbbells slightly wider than shoulder-width apart. Grasp dumbbells.

Extend your legs so that your feet are together. Your arms should be straight down from your shoulders. Do not lock your elbows.

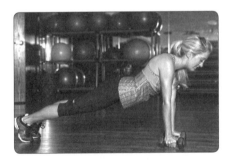 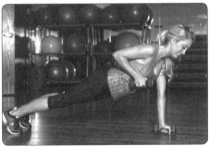

Pull the right dumbbell off the floor, keeping your elbow close to the body. Repeat with the left dumbbell.

Slowly lower your body toward the floor until the elbows form a 90-degree angle.

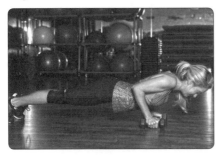

Slowly raise your body back to the starting position, and repeat letters C and D for given number of repetitions.

Note: Go to your knees to make this move easier.

One-arm rear delt fly

On your hands and knees, hold one side of the resistance band in your right hand and grab the other end with your left.

Keep your right hand in place as an anchor as you lift the left arm straight up to shoulder level, leading with your elbow. Squeeze your shoulder blades.

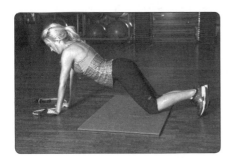
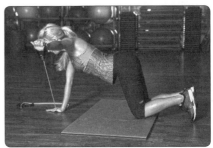

Slowly return to the starting position and repeat for given number of reps before switching sides.

Note: Adjust hand placement to add or decrease tension.

Headbangers

Holding weights, sit on the exercise ball and roll down so that your head, neck, and shoulders are comfortably positioned on the ball. Your knees are bent to form a 90-degree angle, your hips are lifted, and your feet are planted firmly on the floor.

With dumbbells facing each other, extend your arms straight over your chest.

Bend your elbows and lower the weight down to a few inches above your forehead or until your elbows are at 90-degree angles.

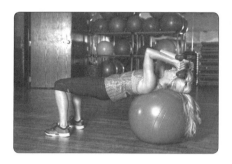 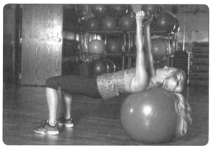

Squeeze your triceps to straighten the arms. Do not lock your elbows.

Ball roll-out

Kneel behind the exercise ball. Lean forward to place your lower arms on the ball.

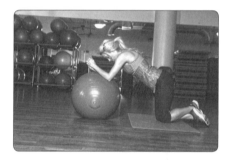 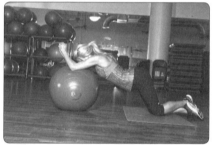

Roll the ball forward by extending your elbows while raising the arms until they frame your head. Don't let your back sag.

Return to the starting position by engaging abdominals.

Circuit 3

Triceps kickback

Holding dumbbells, lie facedown on the ball. Slide your body back slightly so your hips and lower abdomen are on the ball.

Grip the floor with your toes, and open your legs wide enough so you feel stable.

Raise your upper body a few inches so your chest and shoulders rise up and your body forms a diagonal line from your head to heels.

Reach your arms straight out in front of your shoulders with your hands close to the floor.

Bend your elbows and pull your upper arms up behind your back, keeping your arms pinned to your torso, palms facing each other.

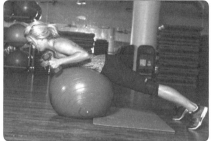

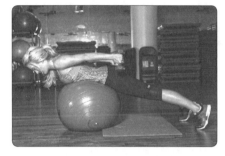

With your elbows bent, extend your arms, squeezing your triceps.

Lower the weights to the starting position.

Hammer curls

Grip each band handle like a hammer. Position your feet hip-width apart on the band.

Keep your abs engaged with your back straight and shoulders back.

Bend your elbows and slowly raise your hands toward your shoulders without rotating the handles.

Slowly reverse the motion and lower your hands back down.

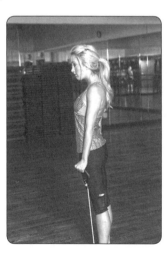 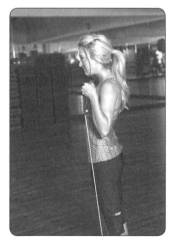

Upright row

Grasp the dumbbells and stand with your feet hip-width apart, palms facing your thighs.

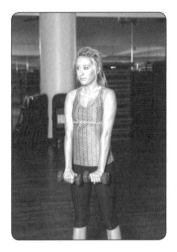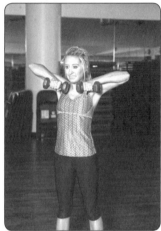

Pull the dumbbells up to your shoulders with your elbows leading out to the sides. Allow your wrists to flex as the weights rise.

Slowly lower and repeat.

Ball side-to-side

Kneel behind the ball, then place your midsection on it. Roll forward until your hands reach the floor.

Walk your hands out until the ball is underneath your knees. Your hands should be shoulder-width apart.

Pike your hips up so your rear points to the ceiling.

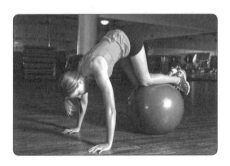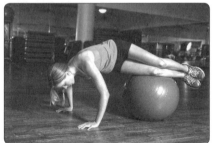

Rotate your hips to the side and bring your knees toward your chest.

Return to the starting position and repeat on the opposite side. Repeat for the given number of reps.

Stretching descriptions

Kneeling chest stretch

Kneel beside the ball. Bend your torso parallel to the floor and place one hand on the top of ball with the palm down. The other hand is on the floor for support.

Press your chest and shoulders toward the floor as the ball provides resistance.

Hold the position and switch sides.

Supine shoulder stretch

Position the ball under your upper back and extend both of your arms out to the side, opening up your chest.

Your feet are shoulder-width apart, and your hips are dropped slightly.

Note: For a greater stretch, allow your hips to drop further.

Bent-over shoulder stretch

Stand behind the exercise ball with your feet slightly wider than shoulder-width apart. Do not lock your knees.

Lower your torso and place the edge of one hand on top of the ball.

Leading with your hand, roll the ball across and to the side of your body.

Hold the position and switch sides.

Bent-over shoulder flexion stretch

Stand with your feet shoulder-width apart.

Bend your torso forward and place your hands on the ball, which is in front of the body.

Roll the ball forward, and hold the position.

Slowly return to the starting position.

Core stretch

Kneel on the floor holding the ball with both hands over your head.

Lean back slightly, and hold the position.

Slowly return to the starting position.

Triceps

Standing, bend your right elbow behind your head and use your left hand to gently pull the right elbow in farther until you feel a stretch in the back of your arm (triceps).

Hold for at least fifteen seconds before switching sides.

Spine twist

Lie on the floor and place your right foot on your left knee.

Using your left hand, gently pull your right knee toward the floor, twisting your spine, keeping your hips and shoulders on the floor, your left arm straight out.

Hold this position for at least fifteen seconds before switching sides.

Circuit 1

Exercise	Equipment Needed	Muscle Groups	Reps
Military press	Pair of light-weight dumbbells, exercise ball	Shoulders, core	15–20
Dumbbell pull-over	One heavy dumbbell, exercise ball	Chest, back, triceps, core, glutes, hamstrings	12–15
Incline chest press	Medium pair of dumbbells, exercise ball	Chest, core	12–15
Single arm lat pull-down	Medium resistance band	Back, biceps	12–15 on each side

Circuit 2

Exercise	Equipment Needed	Muscle Groups	Reps
Dumbbell push-ups with alternating row	Pair of dumbbells (any weight)	Chest, shoulders, back, core	12 push-ups
One-arm rear delt fly	Medium-weight resistance band	Back, shoulders	12–15 on each side

Exercise	Equipment Needed	Muscle Groups	Reps
Headbangers	Pair of light-weight dumbbells, exercise ball	Triceps, core	12–15
Ball roll-out	Exercise ball	Abs, back	10–12

Circuit 3

Exercise	Equipment Needed	Muscle Groups	Reps
Triceps kickback	Pair of light dumbbells, exercise ball	Triceps, core	12–15
Hammer curls	Medium-weight resistance band	Biceps	12–15
Upright row	Medium pair of dumbbells	Shoulders	12–15
Ball side-to-side	Exercise ball	Obliques	6–8 on each side

Note: Remember to cool down.

Stretch	Time
Kneeling chest stretch	15–30 seconds on each arm
Supine shoulder stretch	15–30 seconds
Bent-over shoulder stretch	15–30 seconds on each arm
Bent-over shoulder flexion stretch	15–30 seconds
Core stretch	15–30 seconds
Triceps	15–30 seconds on each arm
Spine twist	15–30 seconds on each side

ROUTINE D

Now that your upper half has been worked and is presently in the process of getting stronger and trimmer, it's only fair to let your legs have a go 'round too! Remember, you'll be performing this routine for three to four weeks in between Routine C. After that, you'll reverse the sequence.

Do the exercises below in the order listed, moving from one exercise to the next without resting. These exercises will not be timed, but you should complete the given number of repetitions as you concentrate on proper form and controlled breathing, exhaling during exertion. Complete the circuit three times before moving on to the next. Rest fifteen to thirty seconds between circuits.

Note: Remember to warm up as you did with the total body routines.

Equipment needed

- Pair of light, medium, and heavy dumbbells

- Exercise ball

- Medium-weight resistance band

- Chair

- Wall

Circuit 1

Lunge on the ball
Holding a dumbbell at either end close to your chest, position your front leg so it is planted firmly on the floor with the foot facing forward.

Step back with the trailing leg and place it on top of the ball with the sole facing up.

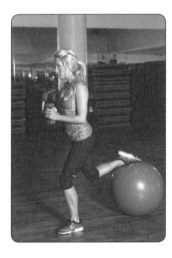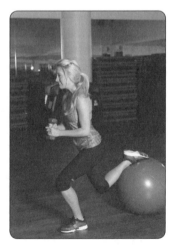

Slowly lower your body straight down. Do not let your knee go past your toe line. (The distance you lower your body will depend on your hip flexibility, but do not go past 90 degrees.)

Return to the start position, and repeat the move for the given number of reps before switching legs.

Ball roll-ins

Lie on your back with your legs extended and your heels on top of the ball.

Press your heels into the ball and lift your hips. Your arms are down at your sides, palms down.

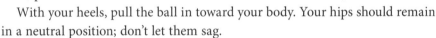

With your heels, pull the ball in toward your body. Your hips should remain in a neutral position; don't let them sag.

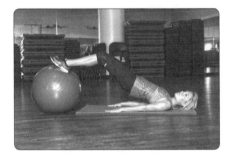 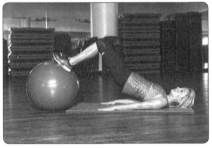

Slowly return to the starting position.

Note: If you feel yourself pushing through your hands, turn palms up.

Plié squat with heel raise

Holding a dumbbell at either end close to your chest, stand with your feet slightly wider than shoulder-width apart. Point your toes outward at a 45-degree angle.

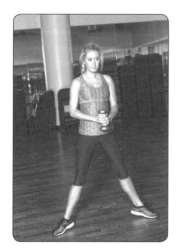
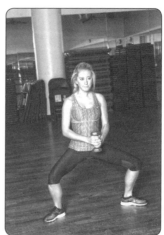

Bend your knees at 90 degrees or as far as you can without compromising good form or losing balance. Keep your hips tucked under and your back slightly arched.

Straighten your legs as you squeeze your rear. As you stand, push up onto the balls of your feet as explosively as possible.

Hold for a second, then lower your heels.

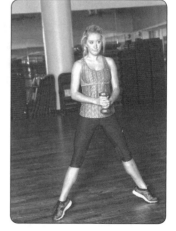

Butt blaster

Get on your hands and knees and wrap the band around the sole of your right shoe. Bend your right knee off the ground. Hold the handles of the resistance band in each hand.

Flex your right foot, and extend your leg straight back, squeezing the glutes.

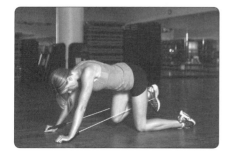
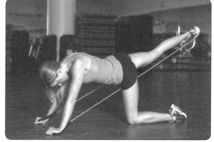

Slowly return to the starting position. Repeat for the given number of reps, then switch to the left leg.

Circuit 2

Squat

Stand on the bands with your feet shoulder-width apart, keeping tension on the band by holding a half-biceps curl.

Lower into a squat, bending your knees to 90 degrees, keeping them behind the toes. Pull on the band to add tension.

Return to starting position.

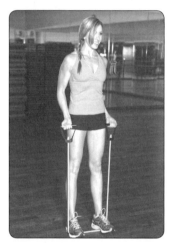 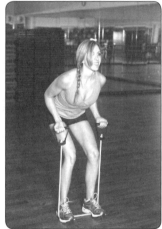

Ball calf raise

Holding the dumbbells, place the exercise ball against the wall, and rest your chest against it.

Using both legs, lift up onto the balls of your feet.

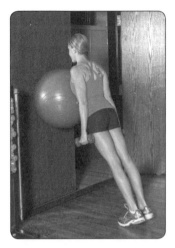 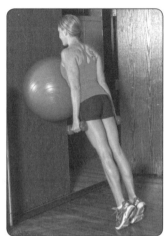

Lower slowly.

Curtsy lunge

Stand with your feet hip-width apart with your hands on your hips.
Take a big step back with your right leg, crossing it behind your left leg.

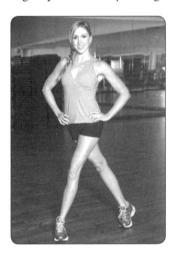 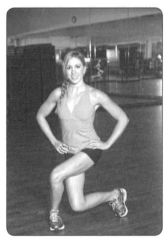

Bend your knees and lower your hips until your left thigh is nearly parallel to the floor. Keep your torso upright and your hips and shoulders square.

Return to the starting position. Repeat for a given number of reps, then switch legs.

Stiff leg dead-lift

Stand with your feet hip-width apart with a dumbbell in each hand.

With your knees straight, lower the weights by bending your hips until your hamstrings are tight or just before your lower back bends.

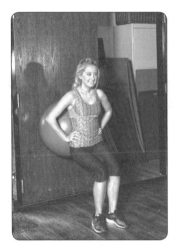 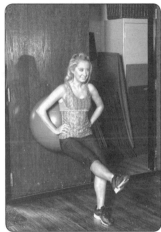

Lift the dumbbells by extending your hips until they're straight.

Pull your shoulders back slightly at the top of the lift.

Circuit 3

Bridge on the ball

Lie on your back with your feet placed on the ball so that your knees are bent. Your hips are slightly off the floor, and your hands are down at your side, palms down.

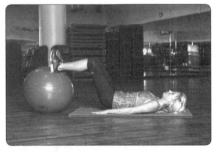

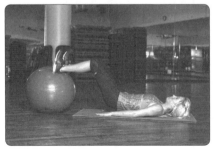

Press down on your feet to lift your hips off the floor. Your hips should stay in a neutral position; don't let them sag, and avoid arching your back.

Gently return to the starting position.

Note: If you find yourself pushing through your hands, turn your palms up.

Ball lift

On a soft surface, place the ball between your feet and lie on your side.

Use the arm on the floor as support for your head. The other hand can be placed on the floor for balance.

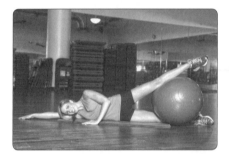 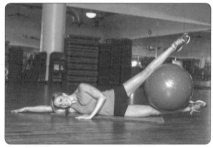

Without moving, squeeze the ball with both feet, lifting the ball off the floor.

Slowly return to the starting position. Repeat for a given number of reps before switching sides.

Squat with leg extension

Place the exercise ball on the wall, positioning it on the mid-lower part of your back. Place your hands on your hips.

Lean against the ball slightly and bend your knees, lowering your body until your knees are at a 90-degree angle.

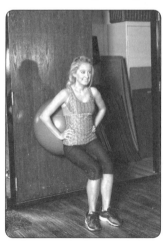 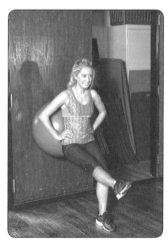

At the bottom of the movement, extend one leg.

Hold and lower the leg, pushing back to the starting position.

Alternate legs with each repetition.

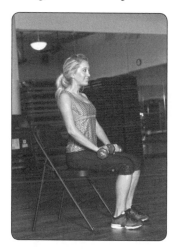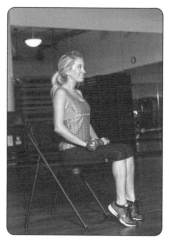

Seated calf raise

Sitting on a chair, hold the dumbbells across your thighs. Sit up straight with your feet flat on the ground.

Lift up onto the balls of your feet, flexing your calf muscles.

Hold this position, and squeeze for 1 to 2 seconds.

Lower your heels to the floor.

Stretching descriptions

Lunge stretch

Straddle the exercise ball, staying centered on it.

Press your back thighs into the ball, causing your hips to tilt backward. The ball will roll slightly forward.

Hold and switch sides.

Bent-over inner thigh stretch

Place the ball to your side. Place your foot on top of the ball.

Roll your foot out to the side to straighten your leg. The knee supporting you should be slighting bent.

Hold and switch sides.

Hips/glutes

Cross your left foot over your right knee.

Grasp your hands behind your right thigh and gently pull your thigh toward you, keeping the body relaxed.

Hold this position for at least fifteen seconds before switching sides.

Inner thigh

Sit on the floor with your feet pressed together.

Keep your abs pulled in as you lean forward.

Keep leaning until you feel a nice stretch in your inner thighs.

Hamstrings

Sit on the floor and extend one leg out straight.

Bend the other leg at the knee, and position the sole of that foot against your opposite inner thigh.

Extend your arms and reach forward over the straight leg by bending at the waist as far as possible.

Hold and switch legs.

Calves

Place both your hands on a wall with your arms extended.

Lean against the wall with one leg bent forward and the other leg extended back with your knee straight and your foot positioned directly forward.

Press your rear heel into the floor, and move your hips slightly forward.

Hold and repeat on the other leg.

Spine twist

Lie on the floor and place your right foot on left knee.

Using your left hand, gently pull your right knee toward the floor, twisting your spine, keeping your hips and shoulders on the floor, with your left arm straight out.

Hold for at least fifteen seconds before switching sides.

Circuit 1

Exercise	Equipment Needed	Muscle Groups	Reps
Lunge on the ball	One heavy dumbbell, exercise ball	Glutes, thighs	12–15 on each leg
Ball roll-ins	Exercise ball	Hamstrings	12–15
Plié squat with heel raise	One heavy dumbbell	Glutes, inner and outer thighs, calves	12–15
Butt blaster	Medium-weight resistance band	Glutes	12–15 on each side

Circuit 2

Exercise	Equipment Needed	Muscle Groups	Reps
Squat	Medium-weight resistance band	Glutes, thighs	12–15
Ball calf raise	Exercise ball, medium pair of dumbbells	Calves	15–20
Curtsy lunge	Yourself	Glutes, thighs	12–15 each side
Stiff leg dead-lift	Pair of medium dumbbells	Hamstrings, lower back	12–15

Circuit 3

Exercise	Equipment Needed	Muscle Groups	Reps
Bridge on the ball	Exercise ball	Glutes, hamstrings	12–15
Ball lift	Exercise ball	Inner and outer thighs	10–12 on each side
Squat with leg extension	Wall, exercise ball	Glutes, thighs	10–12 on each side
Seated calf raise	Chair, heavy pair of dumbbells	Calves	15–20

Note: Remember to cool down.

Stretch	Time
Lunge stretch	15–30 seconds
Bent-over inner thigh stretch	15–30 seconds on each side
Hips/glutes	15–30 seconds on each side
Inner thighs	15–30 seconds
Hamstrings	15–30 seconds on each side
Calf	15–30 seconds on each side
Spine twist	15–30 seconds on each side

TIME TO HIT THE CLUB! CIRCUIT TRAINING AT THE GYM

While there's no place like home, we all, like Dorothy, wouldn't mind a change of scenery every now and then. If you're a member of a gym, have access to a fitness facility in your apartment or neighborhood, or have a visitor's pass, then follow the yellow brick road to a shining wonderland of fresh, fun fitness equipment!

"Why are machines beneficial?" you might ask. Well, machines facilitate a more controlled motion and provide support that helps prevent injury and makes it easier to maintain proper form. Another plus is that they save time because changing the resistance is much simpler with machines than with free weights, like dumbbells. Free weights, on the other hand, require more balance and coordination. An ideal training program incorporates both machines and free weights in order to equally improve joint stability and gain muscle strength.

In this section we'll be focusing on circuits composed of machines and equipment most of us don't have the space—or funds—to have in our homes. But just because we're moving locales, from our humble home gym to Dumbbell Island, doesn't mean we have to relinquish our exercise balls and resistance bands (because I want to show you totally new exercises, I won't be incorporating them into these circuits); feel free to insert one of the at-home moves into your gym routine. Your friends and fellow weight-lifters will be impressed!

Coming up, I'm going to give you a full-body circuit routine followed by two split-based routines that will efficiently focus on individual muscle groups.

Note: Each of these routines may be done alone or with three friends—one for every exercise! You may include more than three others, in which case make sure the one not occupied with an exercise maintains "active rest" by doing an aerobic move, such as jumping jacks or running in place until the interval is done. I'll be adding optional partner exercises at the end of this chapter.

ROUTINE A

Perform Routine A two to three days a week, making sure you give yourself at least forty-eight hours of rest between workouts. Do this for three to four weeks before graduating to Routines B and C, which will focus on your upper and lower body individually.

Do the exercises below for forty-five seconds each in the order listed, moving from one exercise to the next without resting. Complete the circuit three times before moving on to the next, and only rest if you need to.

Note: Remember to warm up for at least five minutes. Since you're in a gym, hop on a bike or elliptical and get your blood pumpin'!

Circuit 1

Smith machine squat
Load light weights onto either side of the barbell.
Place the barbell across your shoulders behind your neck. Your legs are slightly wider than hip width.

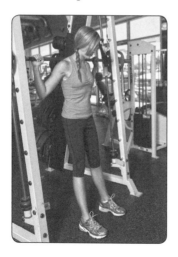 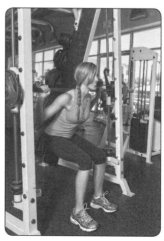

Squat down, pushing your hips back while maintaining a flat back. Your knees should form a 90-degree without jutting out over your toes.

Return to the starting position, pushing through your heels.

Chest press machine

Load enough weight sufficient for a 45-second interval. Adjust the seat so that when you sit, the handles are at shoulder height.

Sit in the machine, pressing back into the pad. Keep your abdominals tight, your shoulders back and down, and your chest up.

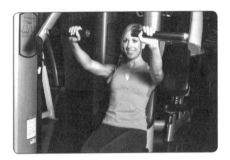 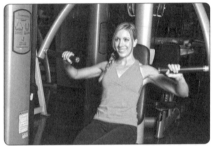

Push the weight out while focusing on bringing your elbows together.

Stop just before your elbows are completely straight and reverse the motion.

Gently lower the weight, stopping when your elbow joints are in line with your shoulders.

Leg extension machine

Load the appropriate weight. Adjust the seat so that the back of your legs are flush with the seat and your back is fully supported.

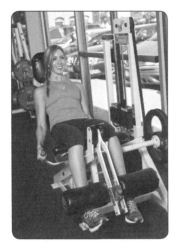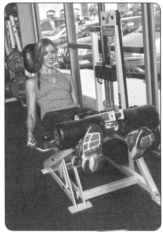

Sit in the machine, placing your feet behind the foot pad. Adjust the foot pad so it rests on your lower shins, above the ankles.

Grasp the handles or put your hands in your lap.

Without flexing your feet and with your abs pulled in, straighten your legs and lift the weight slowly as you exhale. Do not lock your knees.

Hold for one to two seconds, and slowly lower the weight back down—but not completely; the weight stack should not slam.

Cable row

Load the appropriate weight. Sit on the bench, close enough so that you maintain a soft bend in your knees.

Keep your abs tight, your low back arched slightly, and your torso upright.

Lean forward from your hips to grasp the handles and return to an upright position.

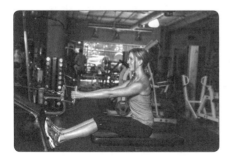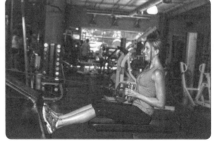

Lower your shoulder blades and row the handles toward your chest, pulling the handles back as far as possible while keeping your arms close to your body. Do not jerk during this movement; row from your upper back.

Slowly allow the arms to extend to return to the starting position.

Circuit 2

Incline leg press

Load the appropriate weight. Adjust the seat so that you don't feel cramped inside the machine.

Sit in the machine with your back and head supported on the seat. Place your feet about hip-width apart on the foot plate. Your knees form a 90-degree angle, in line with the feet. Make sure they don't bow inward or outward.

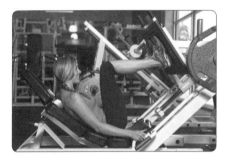 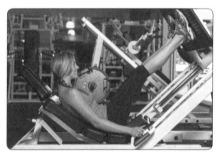

Grasping the assist handles at your side and contracting your abdominals, push the platform away with your heels by extending your knees and hips and pushing your back into the pad. Do not lock your knees.

Slowly return to the starting position.

Decline bench press

Load the appropriate weight. Grab the barbell, and position your hands slightly beyond shoulder-width apart.

Lift the barbell off the rack and slowly lower it until it touches your chest. (Because of the angle of this exercise, it is safe to touch your chest).

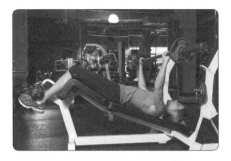 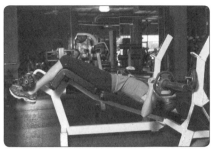

Exhale, pressing the bar up toward the ceiling.

Lying hamstring curl

Load the appropriate weight. Lie facedown on the machine. Position the machine so that the foot pad rests just above your ankles. Grasp the handles below the machine. Place a towel on the machine, and rest your forehead on it to avoid straining your neck.

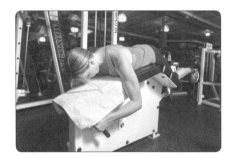 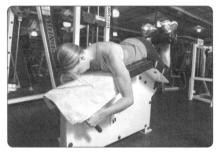

Without jerking, bring your heels toward your buttocks.

In a controlled manner, lower your heels to the starting position without letting the weight slam.

Roman chair knee lift

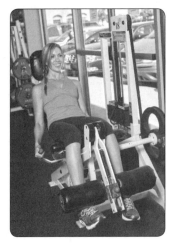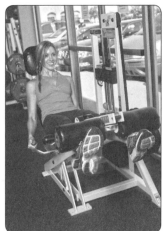

Position yourself so that your back is against the pad and your arms are on the armrests.

Step off the platform so your arms are supporting your weight.

Lift your legs as you bend your knees up toward your chest. Keep your back pressed into the pad.

Slowly straighten your legs as you return to the starting position.

Circuit 3

BOSU squat jump

Note: The BOSU, short for "both sides utilized" or "both sides up," made its debut in 2000 as an innovative training tool that focuses on balance and agility. It resembles an exercise ball that's been cut in half, but to many, it's twice the fun!

Stand on the BOSU with your knees gently bent. Your feet are shoulder-width apart, and your arms are either at your sides or extended out in front of your body.

Slowly lower your body until your thighs are parallel to the floor.

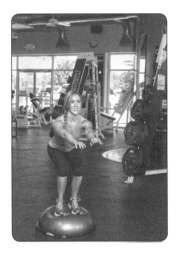 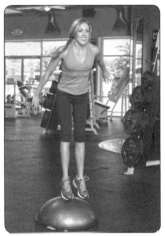

With explosive power, jump straight up. Land on the BOSU softly with your knees slightly bent. Keep abs pulled in to facilitate a soft landing.

Note: To make this harder, try holding a pair of dumbbells at your sides.

Cable flies

Load the appropriate weight to both sides. Position the pulleys so they are at the height of your head.

Stand in the center of the weight stack and grab either handle. Stagger your feet so one is lunged out in front of your body.

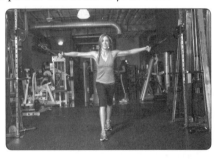

Bend your elbows at a 90-degree angle, and press forward with both arms in a hugging motion. Keep a slight bend in your elbows throughout the movement.

Keep pressing until your hands come close to touching. Hold here for one second, then slowly return to starting position. Do not let the handles go back

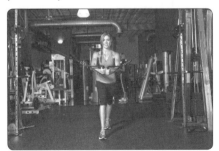

past your shoulders.

Wide grip lat pull-downs

Load the appropriate weight, and adjust the knee pad so it rests on top of your thighs. Grab the bar with an overhand grip just a few inches from the ends.

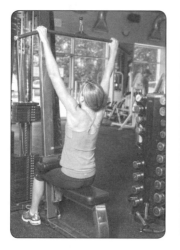 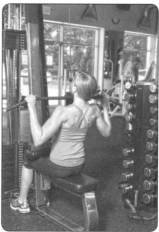

With your chest up, pull the bar down until it is even with your collar bone. Squeeze your shoulder blades together.

Slowly straighten your arms to return to starting position. Do not lock your elbows.

Military press

Load the appropriate weight and adjust the seat so that the handles are at shoulder height.

Sit in the machine with your back pressed into the pad.

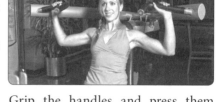

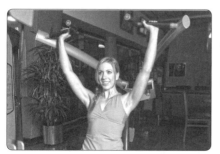

Grip the handles and press them straight up.

Slowly lower the handles so they are even with your shoulders again.

Stretch descriptions

Hips/glutes
Cross your left foot over your right knee.
Grasp your hands behind your right thigh and gently pull your thigh toward you, keeping the body relaxed.
Hold for at least fifteen seconds before switching sides.

Inner thighs
Sit on the floor with your feet pressed together.
Keep your abs pulled in as you lean forward.
Keep leaning until you feel a nice stretch in your inner thighs.

Hamstrings
Lie on the floor with your knees bent.
Straighten one leg up toward the ceiling, and slowly pull it toward you, clasping your hands behind the thigh, calf, or ankle—whichever is most comfy.
Keep your knee slightly bent. Hold for at least fifteen seconds before switching sides.

Chest and shoulders
Standing, interlock your fingers behind your back with your arms straight.
Keeping your hands together, lift them as high as you comfortably can.
Hold the position for at least fifteen seconds.

Upper back
Clasp your hands together in front of your chest with your arms straight.
Round your back toward the floor, pressing your arms away from your body to feel a stretch in your upper back.
Hold the position for at least fifteen seconds.

Triceps
Standing, bend your right elbow behind your head and use your left hand to gently pull the right elbow in farther until you feel a stretch in the back of your arm (triceps).
Hold for at least fifteen seconds before switching sides.

Spine twist
Lie on the floor and place your right foot on left knee.

Using your left hand, gently pull your right knee toward the floor, twisting your spine, keeping your hips and shoulders on the floor, your left arm straight out.

Hold for at least fifteen seconds before switching sides.

Circuit 1

Exercise	Muscle Groups	Time
Smith machine squat	Glutes, thighs	45 seconds
Chest press machine	Chest, triceps	45 seconds
Leg extension machine	Thighs	45 seconds
Cable row	Back, biceps	45 seconds

Circuit 2

Exercise	Muscle Groups	Time
Incline leg press	Glutes, thighs	45 seconds
Decline bench press	Chest, triceps	45 seconds
Lying hamstring curl	Hamstrings	45 seconds
Roman chair knee-lift	Lower abs	45 seconds

Circuit 3

Exercise	Muscle Groups	Time
BOSU squat jump	Thighs, glutes, abs	45 seconds
Cable flies	Chest	45 seconds
Wide grip lat pull-downs	Back, shoulders, biceps	45 seconds
Military press	Shoulders	45 seconds

Note: Remember to cool down before stretching.

Stretch	Time
Hips/glutes	15–30 seconds on each leg
Inner thighs	15–30 seconds
Hamstrings	15–30 seconds on each leg
Chest and shoulders	15–30 seconds
Upper back	15–30 seconds

Stretch	Time
Triceps	15–30 seconds on each arm
Spine twist	15–30 seconds on each side

Routine B

Time to shake and split things up. In this routine we'll focus only on our upper body.

Perform Routine B two days a week and Routine C one day a week for three to four weeks. Then reverse the sequence for another three to four weeks so Routine C is done twice and B once. For example:

Weeks 1–4	Routine	Weeks 5–8	Routine
Monday	B	Monday	C
Wednesday	C	Wednesday	B
Friday	B	Friday	C

After two months, return to the total body format presented in Routine A, making sure you increase resistance and/or the number of repetitions to maintain progress and prevent a plateau.

Do the exercises below for forty-five seconds each in the order listed, moving from one exercise to the next without resting. Complete the circuit three times before moving on to the next, and rest fifteen to thirty seconds between circuits.

Note: Remember to warm up for at least five minutes.

Circuit 1

Barbell bench press
Load the appropriate weight, and lie faceup on the flat bench.

Grab the barbell above you with an overhand grip slightly wider than shoulder width.

Lift the bar off the rack, and slowly lower it until the bar hovers two or three inches above your chest.

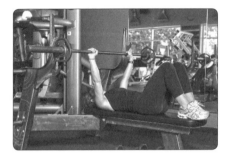 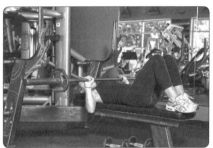

Pause, then explosively push the barbell back up. Do not lock your elbows at the top of the motion.

Assisted wide-grip pull-up

Load the appropriate *assisting* weight. (For this machine, increase the weight to make the exercise easier.) Step onto the step, and firmly grasp the handles so your hands are wide, gripping the bent part of the handles.

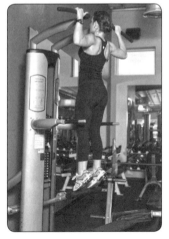

Place your knees, one at a time, on the padded knee rest. You may also stand on the knee rest, if you prefer.

Pull up as far as you can, engaging your abs, keeping your body in a flat line. Squeeze your shoulder blades together. Pause at the top of the movement.

Lower yourself slowly so that arms are nearly fully extended.

Cable curls

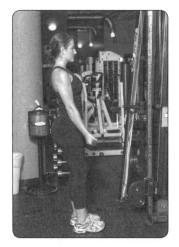 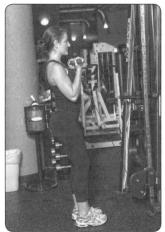

Load the appropriate weight. Grasp the low pulley cable bar with an underhand grip so hands are shoulder-width apart. Stand close to the pulley with your feet hip-width apart and your knees slightly bent.

With your elbows at your sides, curl the bar up until your forearms are vertical. Squeeze your biceps at the top of the motion.

Slowly release the bar back down.

BOSU side plank

Place one elbow the on domed surface of the BOSU. (The flat side of the BOSU should be flat on the ground.) With your body in a straight line from head to toe, lift your hips off the ground. Place your resting hand on your lifted hip.

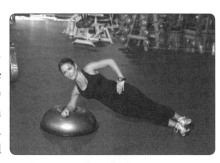

Hold the position for twenty seconds, then switch sides for the duration of the interval.

Circuit 2

Incline dumbbell fly
Holding a pair of dumbbells, lie faceup on an incline bench.

Hold the weights straight above you, palms facing each other, as you press your back firmly into the pad.

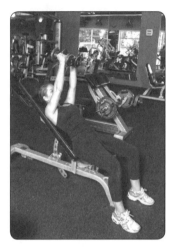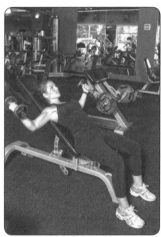

Lower the weights in an arcing motion with your arms wide. Keep a soft bend in your elbows.

Stop lowering once the weights are even with your chest.

Focusing on using only your chest muscles, raise the dumbbells back to starting position. Squeeze your chest muscles at the top of the movement.

Dumbbell row

Place one knee on the bench and the other on the floor for support. Hold the dumbbell in the hand opposite the knee on the bench. (Your free arm helps support on the bench.)

Bend over so that your back is parallel to the ground.

Fully extend the arm holding the dumbbell with your palm facing inward.

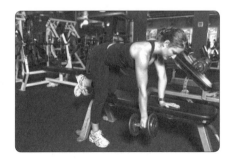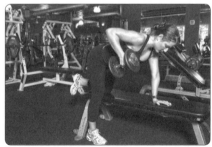

Pull the dumbbell up to your side until it makes contact with or nearly touches your rib cage.

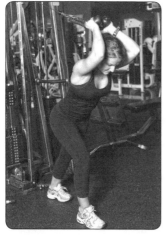

Return to the starting position until the arm is extended and your shoulder is stretched forward.

Cable overhead triceps extension

Clip the rope attachment onto the middle part of the cable machine, and load the appropriate weight.

Grasp either end of the rope's handles, and then lunge one foot out away from the machine, bending forward at your waist.

With your hands above your head, slowly extend your arms until they are parallel to the floor. Do not lock your elbows.

Keeping your upper arms still, bring the rope back until it is above your head.

Decline sit-up with medicine ball

Holding a light- or medium-weight medicine ball, sit on a decline bench, and place your feet under the pad. Slowly lie back onto the bench, but don't allow your shoulder blades to touch the bench.

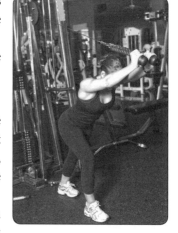

Keeping the ball close to your chest or held in front away from your torso, raise yourself back up until your upper body is vertical.

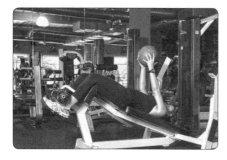 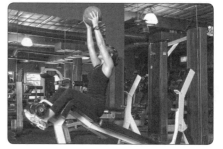

Slowly lower down again, being sure not to let your shoulder blades and neck rest on the bench.

Circuit 3

BOSU push-up

Place the BOSU dome-side down on the ground. Just like in a standard push-up, begin with your legs extended and your toes on the ground (or knees on the ground for a modified version). Make sure your back is straight.

Place your hands on either edge of the BOSU.

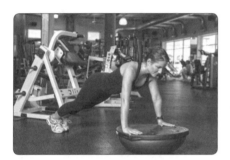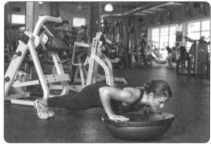

Slowly lower, bending your arms until they are at 90 degrees or until your chest nearly touches the BOSU.

Slowly push back up to the starting position, exhaling as you push.

Rear delt fly on machine

Load the appropriate weight and adjust the handles so they're as close as they can be to the machine. If necessary, adjust the seat so the handles are at shoulder height. Sit in the machine facing the upright pad.

Pull your shoulder blades down, then grasp handles.

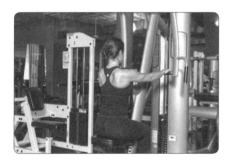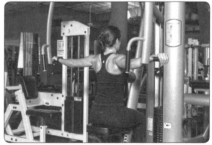

Pull the handles behind your back, squeezing your shoulder blades together. Slowly close the handles as you return to the starting position.

Assisted triceps dip

Load the appropriate weight. (Remember, the more weight you add, the easier the exercise will be.)

Grasp the handles, then step onto bar or foot pads. Place your knees, one at a time, onto the knee pad. You may stand on the bar, if you prefer.

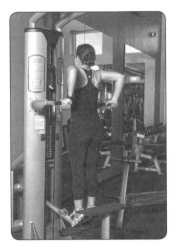 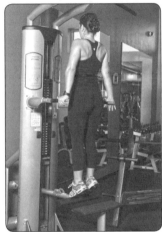

Keeping your abs tight, bend your elbows to lower your body until your elbows are bent at 90 degrees.

Straighten your elbows as you push back up to the starting position, squeezing your triceps at the top of the movement.

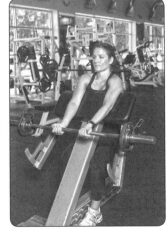

Preacher curls

Adjust the seat of the preacher bench so your underarms rest near the top of the pad. Load the appropriate weight, using just the curl bar if necessary.

Grasp the curl bar with an underhand grip with your hands about shoulder-width apart.

Raise the bar until your forearms are vertical.

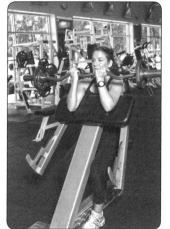

Lower the curl bar until your arms are almost completely extended, maintaining a slight bend in your elbows.

Stretching descriptions

Kneeling chest stretch

Kneel beside the exercise ball. Bend your torso so that it is parallel to the floor, and place your hand on top of ball with the palm down. Your other hand is on the floor for support.

Press your chest and shoulders toward the floor as the ball provides resistance.

Hold and switch sides.

Supine shoulder stretch

Position the exercise ball under your upper back, and extend both arms out to the sides, opening up the chest.

Your feet are shoulder-width apart, and hips are dropped slightly.

Note: For a greater stretch, allow the hips to drop farther.

Bent-over shoulder stretch

Stand behind the ball with your feet slightly wider than shoulder-width apart. Do not lock your knees.

Lower your torso and place the edge of one hand on top of the ball.

Leading with your hand, roll the ball across and to the side of your body.

Hold and switch sides.

Bent-over shoulder flexion stretch

Stand with your feet shoulder-width apart facing the exercise ball (on the floor).

Bend your torso forward and place your hands on the ball.

Roll the ball forward, and hold the position.

Slowly return to the starting position.

Core stretch

Kneel on the floor holding the ball over your head with both hands.

Lean back slightly and hold.

Slowly return to the starting position.

Triceps

Standing, bend your right elbow behind your head, and use your left hand to gently pull the right elbow in further until you feel a stretch in the back of your arm (triceps).

Hold for at least fifteen seconds before switching sides.

Spine twist

Lie on the floor and place your right foot on your left knee.

Using your left hand, gently pull your right knee toward the floor, twisting your spine, keeping hips and shoulders on the floor, with your left arm straight out.

Hold for at least fifteen seconds before switching sides.

Circuit 1

Exercise	Muscle Groups	Time
Barbell bench press	Chest, triceps	45 seconds
Assisted wide-grip pull-up	Back	45 seconds
Cable curls	Biceps	45 seconds
BOSU side plank	Obliques	20 seconds on each side

Circuit 2

Exercise	Muscle Groups	Time
Incline dumbbell fly	Chest	45 seconds
Dumbbell row	Back, biceps	45 seconds
Cable overhead triceps extension	Triceps	45 seconds
Decline sit-up with medicine ball	Upper abs	45 seconds

Circuit 3

Exercise	Muscle Groups	Time
BOSU push-up	Chest, triceps	45 seconds
Rear delt fly on machine	Upper back	45 seconds
Assisted triceps dip	Triceps	45 seconds
Preacher curls	Biceps	45 seconds

Note: Remember to cool down before stretching.

Stretch	Time
Kneeling chest stretch	15–30 seconds on each arm
Supine shoulder stretch	15–30 seconds
Bent-over shoulder stretch	15–30 seconds on each arm
Bent-over shoulder flexion stretch	15–30 seconds
Core stretch	15–30 seconds
Triceps	15–30 seconds on each arm
Spine twist	15–30 seconds on each side

ROUTINE C

I bet your legs are just begging for quality one-on-one time with all kinds of thigh-friendly and literally uplifting machines. The wait is over! In this routine, we'll dive into some of the very best leg exercises fancy gyms have to offer.

Do the exercises below for forty-five seconds each in the order listed, moving from one exercise to the next without resting. Complete the circuit three times before moving on to the next, and rest fifteen to thirty seconds between circuits.

Note: Remember to warm up for at least five minutes.

Circuit 1

BOSU lateral lunge
Turn the BOSU so that it is flat-side down. Hold a light- to medium-weight dumbbell in each hand, and stand about two feet away from the BOSU.

With the leg closest to the BOSU, step to the side, inhaling as you slowly sit back into a lunge with your lead foot on top of the BOSU dome. The other leg is slightly bent.

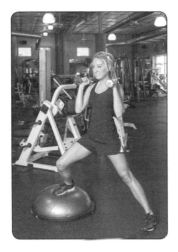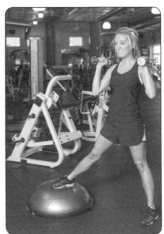

Keeping your weight on the heel of your lunging leg, pause, then exhale as you straighten the lunging leg to starting position.

Repeat for roughly half the time of the interval, then switch legs.

Note: Do not use weights if you find this exercise too challenging.

Dumbbell step-up

Grasp both dumbbells and stand facing a step box or flat bench.

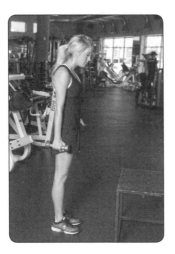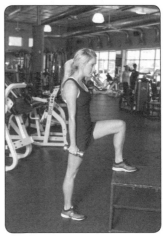

Place the foot of the first leg you will be working on the bench.

Keeping your torso straight and your knee aligned directly over your toes,

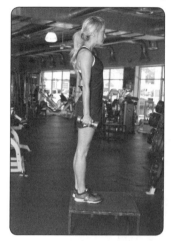

press through your heel to lift yourself onto the bench, bringing your opposite foot onto the bench as well.

With control, lower yourself by stepping down with the foot you stepped up with.

Alternate and repeat.

Smith machine plié squat

Load the appropriate weight on the machine, using only the bar if necessary. Lift the bar, placing it across your shoulders behind your neck, and walk your feet out. Then turn your toes and ankles outward to form a plié stance.

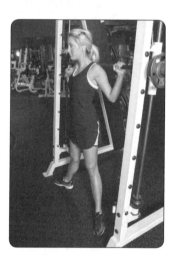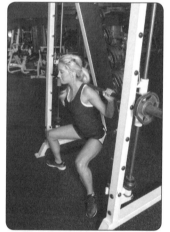

Keeping your back straight and your knees in line with your toes, lower yourself until your thighs are parallel to the ground.

Press through your heels to lift yourself to starting position.

Standing calf raise machine

Load the appropriate weight onto the machine, and adjust the shoulder pads to fit your height.

Step into the machine, placing the balls of your feet on the foot block and your shoulders under the shoulder pads. Your toes point forward.

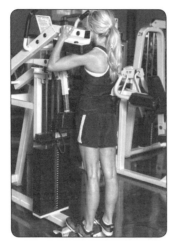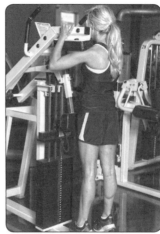

Begin with your heels pointing down, making a nice stretch through your calf muscles. Keep your knees stiff and straight but not locked.

Moving only at your ankles, lift up onto the balls of your feet and squeeze.

Slowly lower to starting position.

Circuit 2

Leg press

Load the appropriate weight on the machine, and adjust the seat if necessary so that your knees are at 90 degrees when you sit in the machine with feet on the foot plate.

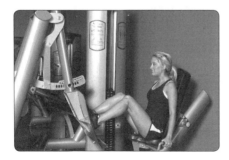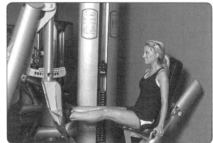

Sit in the machine with your back and head pressed into the pad.

Position your feet about hip-width apart on the foot plate. Your knees are in line with your feet. Make sure they don't bow inward or outward.

Keeping your abs tight and grasping the handles, push the platform away by pressing through your heels. Do not lock your knees.

Return to the starting position by gently allowing your knees to bend.

BOSU stiff leg dead lift

Place the BOSU flat-side down on the ground. Holding either a barbell or pair of dumbbells, step onto the dome of the BOSU, and position your feet in its center about hip-width apart.

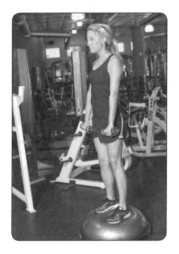 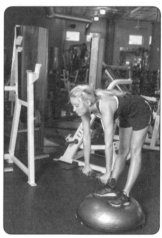

Keeping your abs tight and your knees straight, lower the weights or barbell by bending your hips until your hamstrings are tight, or just before your lower back bends.

Lift the weight by extending your hips until they're straight.

Pull your shoulders back slightly at the top of the lift.

One-legged squat with cable

Attach the rope apparatus to the center of pulley machine, and place the weight stack pin at heaviest weight (solely for support).

Facing the machine, stand about two feet away with your lead foot in the exact center, perpendicular to the machine.

Grasping either end of the rope, lift the foot that is not leading off the ground.

With the lead foot, slowly sit back into a squat. Use the rope only for balance.

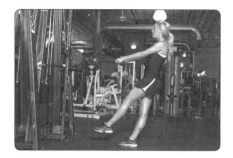 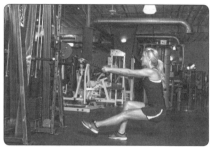

Lower yourself until your thigh is parallel to the floor. Then, pushing with your heel, return to the starting position.

Repeat for half of the interval, and then switch legs.

Calf raises on incline leg press

Load the appropriate weight on the machine.

Sit in the machine with your back pressed comfortably into the pad. Place your feet on the platform hip-width apart.

Unlock the machine and push the platform away using your heels.

Walk each foot to the bottom of the platform so that your toes and the balls of your feet push into the platform.

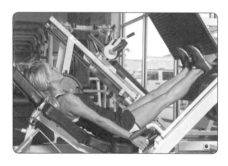 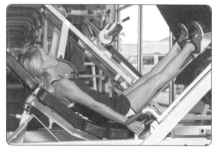

Push the platform by extending your ankles as far as possible, squeezing your calf muscles.

Return to the starting position by bending your ankles. Keep your knees bent slightly throughout the exercise.

Circuit 3

Hack squat machine

Load the appropriate weight. Position yourself in the machine with your back pressed into the pad. Your feet are slightly wider than shoulder-width apart.

Slowly lower yourself as if squatting into a chair. Keep your back flat throughout the movement.

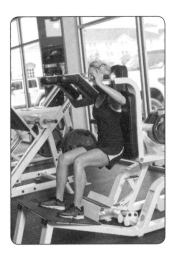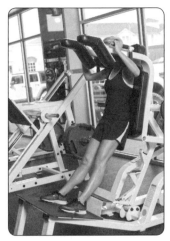

Stop lowering yourself when your thighs are parallel to the ground. Then return to the starting position.

Seated hamstring curl

Load the appropriate weight and adjust the foot pad so it rests below the lower part of your leg, just above your heels.

Press your back into the back pad and grasp the handles.

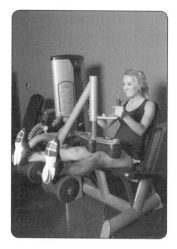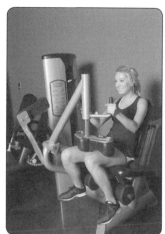

Using your hamstrings and with flexed feet, lower the weight down as if to touch your heels to your hamstrings.

Keeping your feet flexed, slowly return the weight to the starting position.

BOSU lunge

Place the BOSU flat-side down on the floor. With or without dumbbells, stand lunge distance away from the center of the BOSU dome.

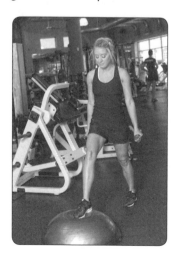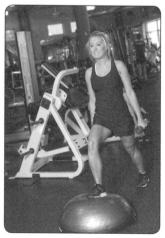

Place your leading foot in the middle of the BOSU dome, then lower into a lunge, keeping your back straight and your knee directly over the ankle placed on the dome.

As you stand, push off the BOSU and step back, bringing your feet together. Switch sides and repeat.

Seated calf raise machine
Load the appropriate weight and sit in the machine. Adjust the seat, if necessary, so the pad rests firmly on top of your knees.

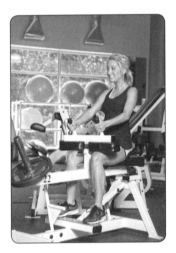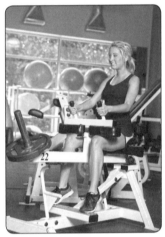

Place your toes and the balls of your feet on the platform. Then press them into the platform, bringing your ankles up as high as you can so you are on your tiptoes.

Return to the starting position.

Stretching descriptions

Lunge stretch
Straddle the ball, staying centered on it.

Press the back of your thighs into the ball, causing your hips to tilt backward. The ball will roll slightly forward.

Hold and switch sides.

Bent-over inner thigh stretch
Place the ball to your side. Place one foot on top of the ball.

Roll your foot out to the side to straighten your leg. (The knee supporting you should be slighting bent.)

Hold this position and switch sides.

Hips/glutes

Cross your left foot over your right knee.

Grasp your hands behind your right thigh and gently pull the thigh toward you, keeping your body relaxed.

Hold this position for at least fifteen seconds before switching sides.

Inner thighs

Sit on the floor with your feet pressed together.

Keep your abs pulled in as you lean forward.

Keep leaning until you feel a nice stretch in your inner thighs.

Hamstrings

Sit on the floor and extend one leg out straight.

Bend the other leg at the knee, and position the sole of that foot against your opposite inner thigh.

Extend your arms and reach forward over the straight leg by bending at the waist as far as possible.

Hold and switch legs.

Calves

Place both hands on wall with your arms extended.

Lean against the wall with one leg bent forward and other leg extended back with your knee straight and your foot positioned directly forward.

Press your rear heel into the floor, and move your hips slightly forward.

Hold and repeat on the other leg.

Spine twist

Lie on the floor and place your right foot on your left knee.

Using your left hand, gently pull your right knee toward the floor, twisting your spine, keeping your hips and shoulders on the floor, with your left arm straight out.

Hold for at least fifteen seconds before switching sides.

Circuit 1

Exercise	Muscle Groups	Time
BOSU lateral lunge	Glutes, thighs	Approx. 22 seconds on each leg
Dumbbell step-up	Glutes, thighs	45 seconds
Smith machine plié squat	Inner thighs	45 seconds
Standing calf raise machine	Calves	45 seconds

Circuit 2

Exercise	Muscle Groups	Time
Leg press	Thighs	45 seconds
BOSU stiff leg dead-lift	Hamstrings, lower back	45 seconds
One-legged squat with cable	Glutes, thighs	Approx. 22 seconds on each leg
Calf raises on incline leg press	Calves	45 seconds

Circuit 3

Exercise	Muscle Groups	Time
Hack squat machine	Thighs, glutes, abs	45 seconds
Seated hamstring curl	Hamstrings	45 seconds
BOSU lunge	Glutes, thighs	45 seconds
Seated calf raise machine	Calves	45 seconds

Note: Remember to cool down.

Stretch	Time
Lunge stretch	15–30 seconds
Bent-over inner thigh stretch	15–30 seconds on each side
Hips/glutes	15–30 seconds on each side
Inner thighs	15–30 seconds
Hamstrings	15–30 seconds on each side
Calf	15–30 each side
Spine twist	15–30 seconds on each side

OPTIONAL EXERCISES WITH PARTNERS

In any of the circuit routines, insert one of the following partner exercises to add a healthy dose of moral support as you trim and tone in tandem. Or if you wish, substitute two of the exercises in a circuit with one it takes two to do! Just make sure the exercise corresponds with the focus of your routine that day.

Exercise	Muscle Groups	Time
Ball toss	Rectus abdominis (the "six pack" muscle)	45 seconds
Exercise ball push	Obliques	45 seconds
V's	Shoulders, upper back	45 seconds
BOSU toss	Obliques	Approx. 22 seconds on each side
Mid-row	Back, glutes, thighs	45 seconds
Kneeling twist	Obliques	45 seconds
Squat with chest pass	Glutes, thighs, chest	45 seconds
Floor slams	Shoulders, abs	45 seconds
Lunge with chest pass	Glutes, thighs, chest	45 seconds

Ball toss

Grab a medium or heavy medicine ball and sit facing one another with toes touching and knees bent.

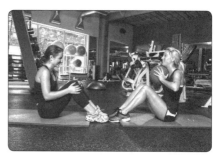

The partner with the ball holds the ball close to her chest, then passes it to her partner, who catches the ball while lying backward. She continues lying backward, stopping before her shoulder blades touch the floor.

The partner with the ball then sits up and tosses the ball to her partner. Repeat.

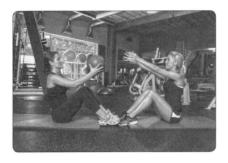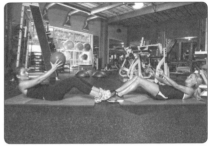

Exercise ball push

Grab an exercise ball and lie down side by side so you're about a foot apart.

Extend your legs up so they're perpendicular to the floor with your feet toward the ceiling. Your head, shoulders, and back remain on the floor.

Place the ball between each of your feet so it touches partner one's inner foot and partner two's outer foot.

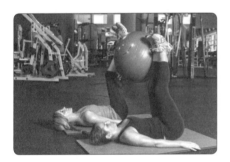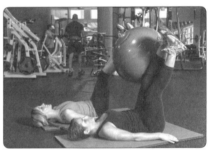

Partner one pushes the ball gently in the direction of partner two, while partner two resists, barely allowing the ball to arc in her direction.

Partner two then reverses the motion, pushing the ball in partner one's direction.

Note: It's very important that both partners maintain pressure on the ball throughout the exercise by engaging your oblique muscles.

V's

Grab two light or medium resistance bands and crisscross them so they form an X. Back up so you're about six feet apart. Grasp a handle in each hand, keeping your elbows and knees softly bent.

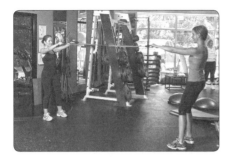 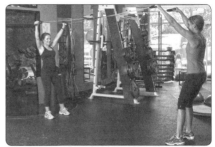

At the same time, raise your arms overhead, forming the shape of a *V.* Squeeze your shoulder blades together.

Slowly return to the starting position.

BOSU toss

Find two BOSUs and position them three to four feet apart with the flat side down.

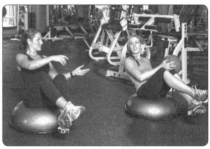

Grab one light medicine ball. Then each of you sit on a BOSU, facing the same direction.

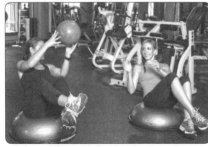

Engaging your lower abs, bend your knees and lift your feet off the ground.

The partner with the ball twists, passing the ball to her partner.

This partner catches the ball, then reverses the motion.

Repeat for about 22 seconds, then turn around to work the other side.

Mid-row

Grab two light- or medium-weight resistance bands and intertwine them, holding a handle in each of your hands.

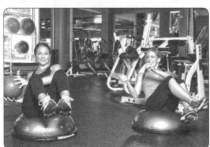

Back up so that you're about six feet apart. Your arms are extended, but the elbow is slightly bent.

With your feet shoulder-width apart, sit into a squat position.

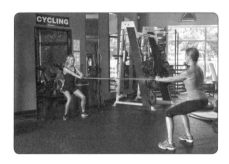 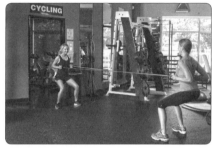

Leading with your elbows, pull the handles back at the same time. Squeeze your shoulder blades together.

Slowly return to starting position, maintaining the squat.

Kneeling twist

Grab a medium or heavy medicine ball and kneel back-to-back with your partner. Keep your abs tight and back straight.

Each of you slowly twist to opposite sides. The partner with the ball hands the ball to the other partner.

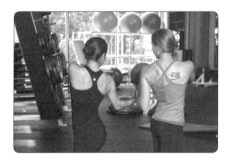 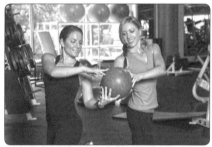

Twist to the other side to pass the ball off again.

Squat with chest pass

Grab a light or medium medicine ball and stand about six feet apart.

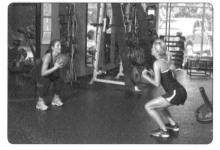

With your feet shoulder-width apart, the partner with the ball sits into a squat position.

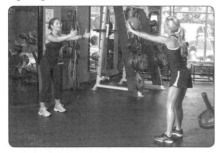

The partner with the ball pushes through her heels to stand up, passing the ball from her chest to her partner.

The partner catches the ball, squats, then rises to pass the ball back.

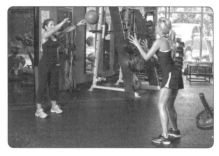

Floor slams

With one partner holding a light medicine ball, stand about six feet apart from each other with your knees slightly bent and your abs pulled in.

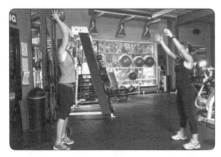

The partner with the ball holds it overhead with her arms extended.

She then bends forward at the waist, using her abs to slam the ball into the ground, passing it to her partner.

The partner catches the ball and repeats the movement.

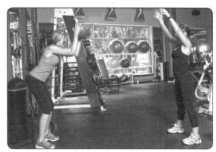

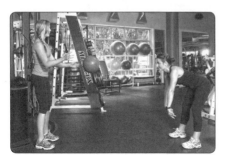

Lunge with chest pass

Grab a light or medium medicine ball and stand about six feet apart.

The partner with the ball lunges forward, passing the ball from her chest to the other partner.

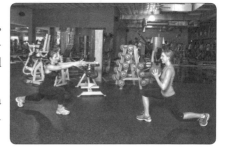

The other partner catches the ball, simultaneously stepping into a backward lunge. She steps into a forward lunge to pass the ball back.

Continue alternating, catching with a backward lunge and passing with a forward lunge.

STRETCHES

Hip/Glute

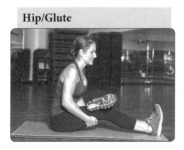

Inner thigh

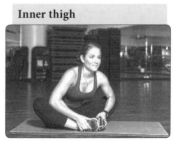

Hamstring

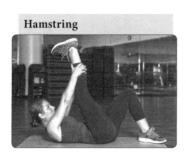

Chest/Shoulders

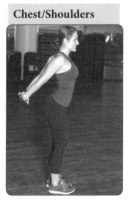

Upper back

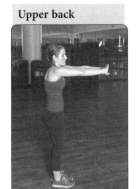

Triceps

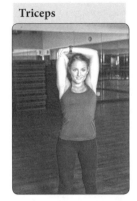

Spine twist

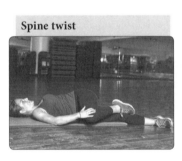

Quad stretch

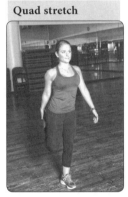

One-arm chest stretch

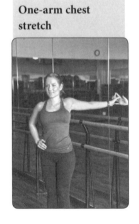

Hamstrings

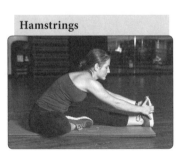

Back extension

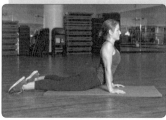 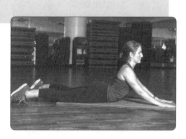

Kneeling chest stretch

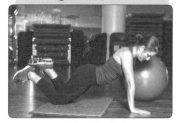 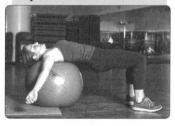

Supine shoulder stretch

Bent-over shoulder stretch

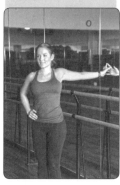

Bent-over shoulder flexion stretch

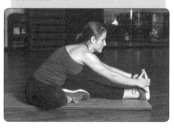

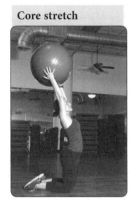

Core stretch

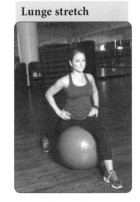

Lunge stretch

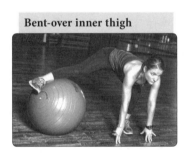

Bent-over inner thigh

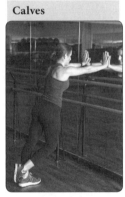

Calves

FITNESS MEETS FELLOWSHIP: CIRCUIT TRAINING WITH FRIENDS

As iron sharpens iron, so one man sharpens another.

—PROVERBS 27:17

Do you ever have a hard time getting out of your jammies and into your Nikes in the morning or feel like you'd rather walk on hot coals than a treadmill for half an hour in the evenings? I know I do! Going to the gym or working out at home doesn't have to be a solo act. In fact, there are a number of reasons to make hitting the weights a social event!

First off, having a partner or small group of workout buddies keeps you committed to a schedule. This accountability goes a long way in helping you maintain your weekly training sessions. I think we'd all agree that it's much easier to cancel on yourself than it is on friends who expect you to show up! Find someone who's willing to commit to a weekly workout appointment with you. By simply knowing you have someone who's expecting you at the gym, track, or Pilates studio, excuses will become fewer and fewer as you become fitter and fitter.

Having the support of a partner or group who notice when you achieve a goal, such as weight loss or when you're able to curl using 10-pound dumbbells instead of 5-pound dumbbells, is a tremendous plus. You'll also stay more focused and attentive as you spot your friend and encourage her to complete a tough set and keep proper form. Such attention to detail will translate into a stellar workout on your part as you correct mistakes and learn to push yourself to new levels of fitness. Most of us have a better time of reaching goals when we have the continual support of someone close to us. Working out is no different!

When I lived in Austin, I worked out for nearly three years with a trainer friend of mine, Colleen. Two or three times a week we met consistently, only canceling if one of us had an emergency situation or a planned trip. There were certainly days when I literally dragged my feet into the gym, wishing I was at home on the sofa and knowing I would be if it were not for my commitment. After only a few minutes into our workout on such uninspiring, *blah* days, my attitude would be totally transformed as Colleen cheered me up simply by speaking words of encouragement and being there for me to lean on, as the song goes. No matter the activity, be it working out with weights or working out a problem in your life, we should all thank the Lord for friends who help us through.

Nowadays I actually instruct a group fitness class. Two mornings a week, women come to the studio, their expressions often conveying very different emotions, ranging from dread and sleepiness to alacrity and effervescence. During the first minutes of class, I marvel as I watch the zombie-like participants snap out of their stupor as they join in with their perkier counterparts. The positive attitudes never fail to banish the negative ones from the room, and everyone leaves an hour later happier, more energized, and revved up for the day. So it is with circuit training with friends: you may not be in the workout mood or zone at first, but being with your fellow fitness fans will make you glad you made the effort.

Fit Fact: According to Debbie Mandel, author of *Addicted to Stress: A Woman's Seven-Step Program to Reclaim Joy and Spontaneity in Life*, a commitment made to exercise keeps you motivated to feel good every day.[3]

7

REMEMBER THE SABBATH

If God Rested, You Should, Too!

For in six days the LORD made the heavens and the earth, the sea, and all that is in them, but he rested on the seventh day. Therefore the LORD blessed the Sabbath day and made it holy.
—EXODUS 20:11

C ONGRATULATIONS, YOU'VE MADE it through the workout pages! Now it's time to take a breather and talk about one of the most important components not only to fitness but also to faith for every believer.

THE SABBATH SHADOW

We're all familiar with the creation story in Genesis. In a theological nutshell, God made the world in six days and rested on the seventh (Gen. 2:2; Exod. 20:11). Please understand, God was not worn out! He simply rested from His work to establish the pattern mankind would later follow. The corresponding Law was given twenty-five hundred years after Creation to Moses on Mount Sinai. It was given not only so the Israelites would reflect on the perfect state of creation and man's relationship with God before sin crept in but also so they would remember their deliverance from the bonds of Egypt.

> Remember that you were slaves in Egypt and that the LORD your God brought you out of there with a mighty hand and an outstretched arm. Therefore the LORD your God has commanded you to observe the Sabbath day.
>
> —DEUTERONOMY 5:15

The Hebrew word for "Sabbath" is *Shabbat*, which means "to rest or to lay aside labor."[1] Every seventh day of the week, Shabbat was to be set apart as a day of rest for God's people. Jesus taught, "The Sabbath was made for man, not man for the Sabbath" (Mark 2:27).

As with the old-covenant sacrifices and ceremonies recorded in the Old Testament, the Sabbath was a picture of something far greater that was to come; it was a precursor to the rest we find in Messiah. The Sabbath is no longer about a religious doctrine to be strictly upheld with tedious rules and rituals and enforced with severe punishment. It is about abiding in the eternal rest provided by Jesus Christ, who came to fulfill the Law (Matt. 5:17). Paul wrote:

> Therefore do not let anyone judge you by what you eat or drink, or with regard to a religious festival, a New Moon celebration or a Sabbath day. These are a shadow of the things that were to come; the reality, however, is found in Christ.
>
> —Colossians 2:16–17

What About Sunday Morning?

Lest we think Christ's fulfillment of the Law nullifies the importance of a weekly church gathering, let's read a key passage found in Hebrews:

> And let us consider how we may spur one another on toward love and good deeds. Let us not give up meeting together, as some are in the habit of doing, but let us encourage one another—and all the more as you see the Day approaching.
>
> —Hebrews 10:24–25

The writer of Hebrews clearly highlights the importance of congregating as followers of Christ. In the first century, it's likely that church membership was dwindling due to fear of imprisonment and even death in Roman arenas. You can be sure there was no such thing as a mega church. In fact, Christians met privately in homes and secret locations to avoid persecution at the hands of those like Saul before his conversion. However, despite understandable fear and rampant persecution, it was important that God's people met together to "exhort" one another.

Ignatius, a student of the apostle John, wrote, "When ye frequently, and in numbers meet together, the powers of Satan are overthrown, and his mischief is neutralized by your likemindedness in the faith."[2] As members of the body of Christ, we are instructed to meet with other believers not only to encourage and be encouraged, not only to worship and listen to an inspiring sermon, but also to bind the "evil spirits in the heavenly places" that seek to scatter and slaughter the sheep of God's pasture (Eph. 6:12, NLT). Just as our natural families provide strength, security, and stability, our local church is our spiritual family, providing protection and blessing as given by our Good Shepherd (Ps. 23:1).

The writer of Hebrews says we are to exhort one another even more as we see the "day" approaching (Heb. 10:25). The "day" he references speaks of Christ's second coming. In can be inferred that Christians today are to be even more exhortative today than the first Christians were! It would appear things have come full circle. The early church was heavily persecuted by the Romans and religious Jews and needed one another's fellowship. As anti-Christian agendas and humanistic worldviews permeate our society, Christians should be pulling together as never before, building one another up as persecution continues to boil in America.

Now you are the body of Christ, and each one of you is a part of it.
—1 CORINTHIANS 12:27

So when did these early Christians meet? It's apparent in Scripture that it wasn't on Saturday, the Jewish Sabbath day. In the Hebrews passage we just examined the writer avoided using the Greek word for "synagogue" when describing the Christians' assembly. (Synagogues, as you may know, are where Jews met on the Sabbath.) In fact, the Greek word from which translators derived "assembling of ourselves together" is *episunagoge*, which is only used one place else in the New Testament to describe the gathering of the saints at Christ's second coming (2 Thess. 2:1).[3]

There are several New Testament passages that tell us the believers gathered on the first day of the week, which is what we know as Sunday (Acts 20:7; 1 Cor. 16:2). This is not a law but rather a tradition that the mainstream churches have maintained for two thousand years. It's unfortunate that injurious divisions have occurred in the church because of a misunderstanding of the Sabbath, some resulting in entirely new denominations! Paul rebuked the Christians in Galatia for returning to such "miserable principles" as the religious Sabbath:

> But now that you know God—or rather are known by God—how is it that you are turning back to those weak and miserable principles? Do you wish to be enslaved by them all over again? You are observing special days and months and seasons and years! I fear for you, that somehow I have wasted my efforts on you.
>
> —GALATIANS 4:9–11

Faith Fact: Jesus performed seven miracles on the Sabbath. The number seven denotes completeness and perfection.

THE RHYME AND REASON FOR REST

You're now perhaps wondering how the old-covenant law of the Sabbath and its emphasis on rest applies to you. Let me tell you! Just as the dietary laws found in the Old Testament were not randomly formulated by our Creator, neither was His notion of an entire day devoted purely to rest.

In the good ol' days, Sundays were set apart in America as a day to rest from work, gather for worship, and enjoy time with family and friends. My mom grew up in the '50s and '60s and can't recall a single restaurant, gas station, or department store ever being open for business on Sunday! My grandmother would cook a lavish Sunday brunch and invite the whole family over after church. They'd spend the entire day simply eating good food, laughing at jokes, sharing stories, and kicking back. My, how times have changed.

Today, Sunday is just an extension of Saturday. Many kids have sporting events on Sundays, teenagers go to the mall and out to eat with friends, countless college kids nurse hangovers and celebrate one more day of weekend, and adults often go in to the office to catch up on paperwork or get a head start on the work week. The concept of rest seems to have become a luxury to be indulged once in a blue moon, not a necessity to enjoy every week.

Rest is important for everything in creation. Here are a few examples:

- Land that is continually worked without being given rest or replenished becomes unfertile.

- If music didn't have spaces of silences and rest, we would only hear noise.

- If our hearts didn't rest between beats, they would stop.

- If various species of animals did not sleep at night, they would get eaten instead.

- If some animals didn't hibernate, they would freeze or starve to death.

Any physician will tell you that rest is essential for good health. When we're deprived of adequate sleep, we put ourselves at risk for sickness and other side effects, such as difficulty concentrating, poor mood, and trouble remembering and thinking clearly.[4] And as fit women, we can negate all the hard work we did in the gym and increase our risks for injury by forgoing much-needed rest.

When I was anorexic, I stubbornly went against the advice of my trainer and worked out for at least an hour, seven days a week. I reasoned I could burn more calories by not taking a day off. Of course, it is true that we do burn calories by working out all seven days, but our bodies become less efficient at recovering and rebuilding when we overwork them. I was, undeniably, overtraining.

Overtraining occurs when a person ignores the body's need to rest, forcing the muscles to remain in a state of damage because they aren't given enough time to repair. Along with my poor diet, overtraining contributed to my constant feeling of lethargy and weakness.

Fit Fact: Our muscles undergo stress during weight lifting or any other intense activity, causing tiny tears. It's during our body's rest that these tears are repaired, resulting in muscle growth.

After I became healthy again, I immediately felt recharged and refreshed each time I stepped into the gym after a day of unadulterated rest. Think of your body as a cell phone; putting it on the charger for a few seconds when the battery is almost dead won't give it very much juice. Likewise, our bodies need ample rest to be totally rejuvenated.

Soul Food

A day should be set aside to rest not only our bodies but also our souls as well. God said through the prophet Isaiah:

> If you keep your feet from breaking the Sabbath and from doing as you please on my holy day, if you call the Sabbath a delight and the Lord's holy day honorable, and if you honor it by not going your own way and not doing as you please or speaking idle words, then you will find your joy in the Lord, and I will cause you to ride on the heights of the land and to feast on the inheritance of your father Jacob.
>
> —Isaiah 58:13–14

I believe this passage reflects the true nature of God's heart for the Sabbath. God desires that we honor Him with one of our most precious possessions—our time. I fear too many Christians go their own way and "speak idle words" every day of the week, never distinguishing a holy day, whether Sunday or another day, to spend with their Creator and Lord. We make our own plans, stay busy, chitchat, go here, go there, keep the TV on, the stereo playing, seldom calling the Sabbath—the laying aside of work—"a delight" or "honorable."

God says that if we draw near to Him, He will draw near to us (James 4:8). The above verse from Isaiah tells us if we honor a Sabbath day, we will find our joy in the Lord. God isn't going to descend into our living room one day a week, take us by the hand, and guide us into a quiet room for some one-on-one time. And we can't leave it up to our preachers to flip on the "Sabbath switch" for thirty minutes a week inside a sanctuary. God longs for us to come to Him personally!

> But when you pray, go into your room, close the door and pray to your Father, who is unseen. Then your Father, who sees what is done in secret, will reward you.
>
> —Matthew 6:6

It's up to us to come to Him for fellowship. God has given us the awesome privilege of entering in His presence, but we must be willing to open the door.

This day of rest is to be a time of physical, spiritual, emotional, and mental renewal. Let's let Jesus be our example. Jesus spent His Saturdays, the Jewish Sabbath day, delighting in God's Word, teaching others, healing the sick, freeing the demonized. He shows us that the Sabbath is no longer a dreaded law to uphold but a joyful day to embrace! Resting from our work, our studies, our obligations, and our workout routines is a God-ordained command given to enrich every fiber of our being. With no time limits, no scheduled appointments, and no pressures, all we're left with is the amazing rest that comes from communing with our Creator.

> Truly my soul waiteth upon God: from him cometh my salvation. He only is my rock and my salvation; he is my defence; I shall not be greatly moved.
>
> —PSALM 62:1–2, KJV

8

A MIGHTY MUSCLE

The Astonishing Power of the Tongue

The tongue has the power of life and death, and
those who love it will eat its fruit.
—PROVERBS 18:21

RICEPS, BICEPS, GLUTES, and quads. Each of these skeletal muscles, along with many more, has been trained sufficiently by now (is anybody sore, yet?), but so far one has been excluded from the fun and games. The most important muscle our bodies possess is a seemingly small one known as the tongue. This four-inch structure contains ten thousand taste buds, which allow us to enjoy all foods—salty, sour, sweet, and bitter.[1] It also, obviously, helps us chew and swallow. A lesser known fact is that our tongues help keep our pearly whites clean! But perhaps the most important function of our tongue is its ability to reach the center of a Tootsie Pop.

Just kidding. Our tongues enable us to talk. But with this awesome gift of communication through speech comes a grave warning label explained in the Bible, one typified by King Solomon in the verse above: the tongue has the ability to bring forth life or death. I believe that when you get a whiff of this wisdom and begin replacing words of negativity, worry, and dread with proclamations of hope, trust, and faith in almighty God, your life will be changed for the better from the inside out.

Say, "Ahh"

I always found it humorous as a little girl when my pediatrician would ask me to stick out my tongue. After all, doing so outside of the doctor's office was a huge no-no that warranted time-out. Now, as an adult, I expect the same question as I saunter into his office and sit on the examination table. No sooner does the doc ask me how I am than he tells me to say, "Ahh," as he examines my throat for anything abnormal.

I now realize that his first question is merely asked for the sake of politeness. In reality, his second request, for me to say, "Ahh," is the one that matters most. His careful evaluation of my throat gives him a fair estimate of my physical condition.

Likewise, the Lord examines my tongue and the fruit it produces to assess my spiritual condition. Many passages address a direct link between our heart and our mouth. In the Gospel of Matthew, Jesus states:

> For out of the overflow of the heart the mouth speaks. The good man brings good things out of the good stored up in him, and the evil man brings evil things out of the evil stored up in him. But I tell you that men will have to give account on the day of judgment for every careless word they have spoken. For by your words you will be acquitted, and by your words you will be condemned.
>
> —Matthew 12:34–37

In essence, if the heart is good, the words will be good, and if the heart is evil, the words will reflect it. Earlier, in Matthew 12 and also in Matthew 7, Jesus compares the heart to a tree. The nature of our "tree" inevitably determines the specimen of "fruit" it produces from our mouths.

Many of us fall into the trap of considering ourselves righteous and good, but the ultimate indicator is the fruit we bear with our lips. In all honesty, I can recall an occasion while driving merrily along a main street near the University of Texas campus in Austin when a woman suddenly rear-ended me. Trust me when I tell you that the first words that escaped my mouth were definitely not PG-rated. I immediately covered my mouth with my hand, completely stunned by what I had shouted.

I had the semblance of wholesomeness and considered myself more pious than your average co-ed, but I quickly realized that external facades are just that, facades. I had drifted from the Lord, not dramatically but ever so slightly. I hadn't been spending time in His Word or in prayer. I wasn't seeking Him or praising Him in worship as in times past. I had allowed myself to be conformed to the pattern of this world and let the peace of God, which guards our hearts and minds, go from me as I strayed from His presence (Rom. 12:2, Phil. 4:6–7).

The apparent involuntary response of my mouth was merely a by-product of the seeds I had planted in my heart. What sprung forth was bitter fruit, perhaps even a rancid vegetable! This wake-up call moved me to repentance as the Holy Spirit whispered, "That is not who you are! You are God's child. Draw near to Me, and you will speak like it!"

> If anyone considers himself religious and yet does not keep a tight rein on his tongue, he deceives himself and his religion is worthless.
> —JAMES 1:26

It doesn't matter how many mission trips you've been on, how many service projects or outreach programs you've been a part of. In themselves, all those things are good, but if we don't keep a "tight rein" on our tongue, our religious deeds are worthless. James goes on in chapter 3 to describe the vital role of our tongues:

> We all stumble in many ways. If anyone is never at fault in what he says, he is a perfect man, able to keep his whole body in check.
> —JAMES 3:2

If we can control our tongue, every other muscle will fall into submission after it. James writes on and equates the tongue with a horse, a biblical symbol of strength. As a former barrel racer, I know just how imperative a bit is when trying to control a fifteen-hundred-pound animal! Just as this diminutive contraption directs a horse, our tiny mouths dictate where our lives go.

All in all, James compares the tongue to the bit of a horse, the rudder of a ship, and the spark that ignites a forest fire. What's the commonality shared by these three? Each instigating object is the smallest component, yet they have the most power and influence to produce incalculable, perhaps even irreparable, damage.

YOU MAKE THE CALL

Like a ship's rudder, our tongue is not immediately seen. We often make a first impression about a person based on her appearance. After she's spoken awhile, however, our impressions can be totally reshaped. I'm sure if someone had seen me moments before I was rear-ended on Guadalupe Street, he would've thought I was a Girl Scout leader by my cross necklace and my Bible still lying in the front seat from church the Sunday before. Seconds later my words would betray the reality of my spiritual condition! Not only do our tongues influence the way we are perceived, but they also determine our destinies.

Let's look at an Old Testament example that makes this point abundantly clear. This incident is found in Numbers 13 and 14 and deals with the Israelites' entry into the Promised Land. They had been liberated from the bonds of Egypt, and it was time to scout out the land God had ordained for them. God instructed Charlton Heston—I mean Moses!—to send twelve men to spy on the land beyond to get a feel for its inhabitants, its cities, and its fruit. These spies spent forty days traversing the land and returned with the report recorded in Numbers 13:26–28:

> They came back to Moses and Aaron and the whole Israelite community at Kadesh in the Desert of Paran. There they reported to them and to the whole assembly and showed them the fruit of the land. They gave Moses this account: "We went into the land to which you sent us, and it does flow with milk and honey! Here is its fruit. But the people who live there are powerful, and the cities are fortified and very large. We even saw descendants of Anak [giants] there."

God had promised His people this land that flowed with "milk and honey," yet ten of the twelve spies injected a big, fat *but* into God's plan. That was a fatal blow that brought tremendous distress and anxiety to the people. Caleb and Joshua, however, had no *buts* about going ahead in the will of God.

Then Caleb silenced the people before Moses and said, "We should go up and take possession of the land, for we can certainly do it." But the men who had gone up with him said, "We can't attack those people; they are stronger than we are."

—NUMBERS 13:30–31

Note the distinct difference between the groups: one said they were able to overcome, the other was resolute they couldn't. As the story continues, we see that each camp ate the fruit of their words. God told the people, "As ye have spoken in mine ears, so will I do to you" (Num. 14:28, ASV). God allowed Caleb and Joshua to enter into the Promised Land while the worrywarts died in the desert.

Lest you think such a tale is inapplicable to your life in the twenty-first century, take a look at a crucial New Testament scripture:

Therefore, since the promise of entering his rest still stands, let us be careful that none of you be found to have fallen short of it. For we also have had the gospel preached to us, just as they did; but the message they heard was of no value to them, because those who heard did not combine it with faith.

—HEBREWS 4:1–2

God still promises a Promised Land for those who choose to follow Him. But before we enter this place of peace and rest, we have to be careful not to fall short of it, as the Israelites did in Moses's day. Despite hearing the message of promise from God, they chose to focus on the tangible signs of danger rather than latch hold of faith in a King greater than their circumstances. The giants and impregnable cities were enough to provoke them to say, "But." Kudos to Caleb and Joshua, who, like King David four hundred years later, saw the formidable foe and still exclaimed, "The battle is the Lord's"!

When you face giants in your life and find yourself in the midst of a situation that seems hopeless and bleak, how will you steer your tongue? Will you allow the horse to run free, or will you pull him back and turn him around? Will you agree with God, who tells us we can do "all things through Christ" who strengthens us, or will you subscribe to the lies of the enemy who tells you it's impossible (Phil. 4:13, KJV)?

Eighty-five percent of the twelve men sent to check out the land refused to trust God. Today, the number of people who choose to assent to the promises of God pale in comparison to the scores of those who allow others and the enemy to supplant God's Word with all kinds of negative assertions.

Let's all repeat after Caleb: "We can certainly do it!"

GOOD WORDS, GREAT FRIENDS

A vocabulary of truth and simplicity will be of service throughout your life.

—WINSTON CHURCHILL[3]

If you've ever experienced the ending of a friendship or gone through a breakup, you can probably think back and recall a time when harsh words were heavily involved in the relationship's demise. For good or ill, our words determine the quality of every relationship we have on this planet. Words are what keep us connected. Whether we're face-to-face in Starbucks, texting from miles away, Facebooking, Tweeting (I can't believe those are verbs!), e-mailing, or using the phone the old-fashioned way, what we say either builds, burns, or repairs bridges.

There have been many times I've been out to eat with a group of girls, some of whom I've just met, and I'm shocked by the derisive tone of the conversations. One might go like this:

Ashley: Erica, I love your purse! It's so cute!

Erica: Thank you. My boyfriend bought it for me.

Hannah: Ashley, if you could ever keep a boyfriend, maybe you'd have that purse too!

Ashley laughs, but a closer look into her eyes would tell you those words wounded her. No matter Hannah's intentions when she commented on Ashley's love life, her tongue wielded a weapon against her friend. It may have been funny to the rest of the table, but to Ashley, the jab was destructive.

I'm sure all of us have been both the victim and the perpetrator in similar situations. It's important to realize the power of our tongues, not just in their operation in our own lives but in the lives of others. The good news is that same weapon of words that drove a wedge through the friendship can be the same instrument that restores it. By confessing you were wrong, whether you realized it at the time or not, and asking for forgiveness, you can encourage your friend while bolstering your relationship with her.

While working out with friends, it is especially critical that you speak affirming words, words that build up and exhort rather than tear down and discourage. If one in your group is not as strong or has a tougher time keeping up, don't sigh loudly, roll your eyes, and with a passive aggressive tone tell her to get with the program. Put yourself in her position. Jesus taught us to treat others the way we'd like to be treated (Matt. 7:12). We all know how we'd like to be treated, but it's another task altogether to bestow that treatment on others. If you find yourself struggling to speak encouraging words, ask the Lord to give you the grace to be uplifting. He tells us in His Word that we shall have whatever we ask for according to His will, and of course, it is always His will for us to speak edifying words to one another.

> Do not let any unwholesome talk come out of your mouths, but only what is helpful for building others up according to their needs, that it may benefit those who listen.
> —Ephesians 4:29

A New Definition of "Bad" Words

Today, when we hear the word *cursing*—or here in Texas, *cussin'*—we generally assume it's describing the four-letter words we hear in PG-13 movies and even prime-time TV. I used to conjure up the fanciful, Hollywood renderings of witches, gypsies, and sorcerers when I heard someone say a curse was brought upon a person or place. With a bit of study into the Word of God, it becomes evident that curses are more than "bad" words and Harry Potter.

In the Bible, cursing doesn't pertain to foul language alone but to the deplorable act of pronouncing a curse upon someone or something. Jesus illustrated this when He and His hungry disciples approached a fig tree on their way to Jerusalem. Seeing the tree had no fruit to offer them, Jesus cursed it, saying, "May you never bear fruit again!" (Matt. 21:19). Immediately the tree withered from the roots up, causing the disciples to "ooh" and "ahh" as you can imagine, yet this was no surprise to Jesus, because He understood the power of words. After His disciples commented, Jesus replied:

> I tell you the truth, if you have faith and do not doubt, not only can you do what was done to the fig tree, but also you can say to this mountain, "Go, throw yourself into the sea," and it will be done. If you believe, you will receive whatever you ask for in prayer.
> —MATTHEW 21:21–22

This is an awesome testament to the power of words, and it came straight from the mouth of our Savior! I hope and pray we can all respect the power we hold in our tongues and use it only to bless. It grieves me to hear people casually toss out the ubiquitous four-letter word *damn* like it's a baseball being pitched in Little League. This is the root word for "damnation" that describes the horrible state of eternal separation from God! In case you need to be reminded, this is the worst possible condition a human being can ever face. God tells us that if we love cursing, it will come to us, whatever it is that we speak (Ps. 109:17). Why would anyone want to damn themselves or anyone else?

Psalm 45 gives a wonderful, prophetic picture of the Messiah and tells us, "Grace is poured into [His] lips" (Ps. 45:2, KJV). His lips, full of grace, are the first things described in this beautiful revelation! If we are to be conformed to the likeness of Christ, shouldn't we strive to have lips like His (Rom. 8:29)? Maybe one day in heaven, we'll all wear grace-flavored ChapStick. I bet its scent would be, well, heavenly!

MIRROR, MIRROR

As American women, not a day passes in which we aren't subjected to a deluge of glitzy movie posters, airbrushed billboards, commercials, and TV shows filled with women Hollywood has labeled beautiful (and most of us would have to agree). With their perfectly styled hair, flawless makeup, spray-on tans, and thin figures, it's no wonder they're paid big bucks to be entertainment starlets. While most of us (I hope!) don't envy many of their self-seeking, decadent lifestyles, it's hard not to desire to at least look like them. It's certainly not harmful to look up to fit, healthy women; I could name a few actresses whom I admire for their disciplined work ethic and clean eating regimens. The danger, however, lies in the propensity to compare ourselves not only to those in the glossy pages of *Us Weekly* but to anyone whose bodies we enviously admire.

Fit Fact: "A study found that 95 percent of women overestimate the size of their hips by 16 percent and their waists by 25 percent, yet the same women were able to correctly estimate the width of a box."[4]

Before my struggle with an eating disorder, just as I was starting to work out, I began to constantly take notice of celebrities and read up on how they attained their sleek physiques. I can recall times I'd stand in front of my bathroom mirror and take inventory of what body parts needed the most attention and which ones were doing OK. I had taken mental photographs of those women I wanted to look like, and until the reflection in my mirror matched those photos, I wouldn't be satisfied.

I'm never going to look like her. My stomach is never going to be that toned. I'd have to eat like a bird to look that lean. All those statements, plus many others, sprung from my lips like weeds on a riverbank. Little did I know that I was pronouncing a curse upon myself and that those toxic words were planting the roots of anorexia that would plague my life in months to come.

I hear many women complain about their appearances. From "flabby triceps" to "thunder thighs," no one seems to have anything good to say about themselves. The good news is, God has plenty of good things to say (Jer. 29:11)! I believe that if we could replace our complaints and curses with praise and thanksgiving, we wouldn't have the physical hang-ups many of us wrestle with. If you find that the last few pounds you need to lose are just "too stubborn to leave" or that your knees just "can't ever seem to feel right" while you work out, think back on how you've been talking. You may have inadvertently placed a curse upon your progress with your own tongue.

So what's the remedy? Praise! Begin praising the Lord for redeeming you, for giving you a second birth by virtue of His Son, for blessing you with gifts, friends, family, and for everything He's done, is doing, and will do in your life. These life-giving words agree with the Word of God and will replace the spirit of dissatisfaction, anxiety, and insecurity with assurance, peace, and confidence. Hebrews 13:15 says, "Through him then let us continually offer up a sacrifice of praise to God, that is, the fruit of lips that acknowledge his name" (ESV). The key word in that verse is "continually." No matter the circumstance, no matter your feeling at the moment, praise God with your lips, and taste the delicious fruit it brings!

BEYOND FLESH AND BLOOD

The Importance of Spiritual Armor

Therefore put on the full armor of God, so that when the day of evil comes, you may be able to stand your ground, and after you have done everything, to stand.
—EPHESIANS 6:13, NKJV

THROUGHOUT THIS BOOK we've learned that we have a great responsibility to take care of our bodies. With our hearts and minds focused on serving God and others, and as we fuel our bodies with healthy, God-made foods and weight train consistently, we see that fitness goes hand in hand with faith as it enables us to live vibrantly for Christ.

In this chapter, we're going to switch gears a bit, moving from the evident and external natural world to the invisible realm of the supernatural—and I'm not talking about *The Twilight Zone*! Now that we've physically equipped ourselves with fit, able, strong, confident bodies, it's time to arm ourselves spiritually. And boy, oh boy, does the Word have a lot to say about it!

"MY BIG FAT GREEK" BATTLE: A TECHNICAL LOOK AT EVERY BELIEVER'S BATTLEFIELD

Do you ever have one of those days where it feels like someone, or perhaps a guerrilla gang, is working behind the scenes of your life to sabotage you, or as if there's an unseen rain cloud hovering ominously above your head, poised to send bolts of lightning at random intervals? Have you ever watched and wondered how Christian speakers and pastors could go from the heights of influence and leadership to the depths of humiliation and shame due to a moral failure? Whether the attack comes through discouragement or temptation, as Christians we each face a common enemy whose purpose is to blind sinners from the truth and dishearten and oppress God's children. That is precisely why we need to understand Satan and his diabolical agenda so we are not "ignorant of his devices" (2 Cor. 2:11, KJV).

The Greek word *methodos* is used in the New Testament to describe Satan's insidious strategies against followers of Christ. *Methodos* literally means "with road."[1] *Methodos* conveys the idea of a traveler on a road. Satan, like anyone going on a planned road trip, knows his destination, and he knows how to get there. When my girlfriends and I have just a few hours on a Thursday afternoon to drive to the outlet mall, we ain't wasting any time on a scenic route! Satan, knowing he has limited time, isn't going to squander any of it driving up and down multiple routes. After thousands of years in the deceiving business, the road is well worn, but it works for him, as history can confirm.

Ready for another Greek lesson? In the verse from 2 Corinthians above, the word for "devices" in Greek is *noemata*, which relates to the word *nous*, meaning "mind" or "intellect."[2] In essence, Paul is saying we aren't ignorant of how the enemy's strategizing mind works. If we put these two ideas together, we get a very astute portrait of the devil, and it isn't the one with a bright red pitchfork and a pointy tail! No, Satan is an exceedingly evil spirit being whose destination is the minds of sinners and Christians alike and whose goal is to confuse, discourage, depress, distress, and tempt those minds.

On to Greek lesson number three. Second Corinthians 10:4–5 says, "For the weapons of our warfare are not carnal but mighty in God for pulling down strongholds, casting down arguments and every high thing that exalts itself against the knowledge of God, bringing every thought into captivity to the obedience of Christ" (NKJV). "The words 'bringing into captivity' are from the Greek word *aichmalotidzo*, which pictured a soldier who has captured an enemy and now leads him into captivity with the point of a sharpened spear thrust into the flesh in his back. "Bringing into captivity" comes from the Greek *aichmalotidzo*, which pictures a soldier who is leading a captured enemy with the point of a spear pushed into his back! The spear point reminds the captured soldier that if he dares escape, that point will be introduced to his insides. Wisely, the captive remains silent and submissive to his captor.[3]

The tense in which Paul writes this verse describes the ongoing action of taking an enemy captive.[4] As believers, we don't deal with Satan once and for all. Yes, he has been defeated at the cross, and we have victory over death through the blood of Jesus, but until Christ returns to crush that old serpent's head or we go to meet Him when we die, there is still a war being waged against us. We are soldiers for a lifetime, and as such, we need to constantly have our spear in hand, ready to direct its point into the back of our enemy. By making mental decisions to cast out every harmful thought planted in our minds and forcing them into submission, we can effectively ward off the flaming darts of the enemy.

No More Damsels in Distress

When I was a little girl, I loved to be read fairy tales at bedtime. *Cinderella* and *Sleeping Beauty* were my favorites. As I got older, I read the tales of King Arthur, Lancelot, and Guinevere and often reenacted Shakespearean vignettes wearing the most medieval-looking dress I could find—often a Disney princess costume. My parents even took me to Renaissance fairs, where I would set out to meet my knight in shining armor at the jousting tournament. Of course, all I found was funnel cake and bad wigs. Yes, it's fair to say I had my head in the clouds!

I'm sure many of you can identify with my wildly romantic notions, and perhaps you, like me, had more than a few crushes on hunky actors who portrayed valiant knights who knew how to treat a lady! I had an innocent fantasy that one day I would be braiding my beautiful, ridiculously long hair in a faraway tower when all of a sudden a dragon would threaten my lofty abode with his fiery breath, and my very own knight, clad in shimmering armor, would come to my rescue. We'd then lope softly into the sunset upon his faithful steed.

If you think about it, as Christian ladies, that fantasy has come true! We were once trapped in our sins (the tower) and headed for hell (the dragon) because of our inherent sin nature. But Christ, the King of kings and Lord of lords (the Knight, of course), came to our rescue, saving us from damnation, freeing us from the bounds of sin, and reconciling us unto God!

But it's not "happily ever after" just yet. We are the bride of Christ, but the wedding banquet has not yet taken place. (Christ isn't done sending out His invitations!) We are still mortal damsels in the line of fire, but we don't have to be in distress. Hallelujah! The Knight we are betrothed to has given us the armor needed to fight until He returns again on that white horse (Rev. 19:11).

Put on the whole armour of God, that ye may be able to stand against the wiles of the devil. For we wrestle not against flesh and blood, but against principalities, against powers, against the rulers of the darkness of this world, against spiritual wickedness in high places. Wherefore take unto you the whole armour of God, that ye may be able to withstand in the evil day, and having done all, to stand. Stand therefore, having your loins girt about with truth, and having on the breastplate of righteousness; And your feet shod with the preparation of the gospel of peace; Above all, taking the shield of faith, wherewith ye shall be able to quench all the fiery darts of the wicked. And take the helmet of salvation, and the sword of the Spirit, which is the word of God.

—EPHESIANS 6:11–17, KJV

We are warrior princesses, even fiercer than Xena! Just look at what our armor consists of:

- Belt of truth
- Breastplate of righteousness
- Shoes of peace
- Shield of faith
- Helmet of salvation
- Sword of the Spirit

Now let's zoom in on each piece individually and learn how we can be ready for attack at all times!

THE BELT OF TRUTH

Before we look at this first piece of armor, it's important to note that twice in Ephesians 6 we are told to "put on" the armor of God, the first time so we might stand against the devil's schemes and again so that we can stand our ground when the day of evil comes. We cannot pick and choose what pieces of armor we'll put on. Have you ever seen a knight in a movie or at a Renaissance fair walking around with his breastplate on but instead of a helmet, a baseball cap, or instead of the proper footwear, a pair of flip-flops? If we choose to omit a single item, we leave a perfect spot for the enemy to paint a bull's-eye.

And also notice this: there is no protection for our backside! The implication is that God's army should be free of deserters! Looking at each of these characteristics, from truth and righteousness all the way down to allegiance and bravery, we can see that this armor is nothing less than Jesus Himself! In writing to the Romans, Paul told them to "put on the Lord Jesus Christ" (Rom. 13:14, NKJV). Each morning as we get dressed, we should also "put on" Christ and wear Him as naturally as we would a sundress. How cool that we can have an invisible layer of supernatural clothing that protects us from evil and deflects the arrows of the enemy!

This belt of truth is an interesting piece to begin with, because it actually has nothing to do with soldier's armor. Belts were worn by most Roman citizens, not just soldiers. These "girdles" were six-inch belts made of linen or leather that fastened around the middle. They were worn outside the long robes commonly worn in the first century. In 1 Peter, we're told to "gird up the loins" of our minds (1 Pet. 1:13, NKJV). Gird up our loins? What on earth does that mean? Well, because their robes were so long, whenever a Roman wanted to move quickly, he'd grab his robe, pull it up, and stuff it into his belt. (No one likes running in a dress.) When a soldier was sent into battle from a garrison, he would do the same thing so He wouldn't trip on his way there.[5]

As Christians daily going into battle, the belt of truth is a key to our preparation. Without securing our belt, we cannot stabilize the bigger pieces of our armor, and the fight becomes cumbersome. Just as the belt is the foundation of our armor, truth is the foundation of our faith. Jesus calls Satan the "father of lies," and as such, deception is his most effective weapon (John 8:44). Without the truth of Jesus Christ, we are defenseless against the falsehoods and half-truths Satan fires our way.

Jesus said, "Then you will know the truth, and the truth will set you free" (John 8:32). We have to know the truth before we can arm ourselves with it. As we discussed in chapter 4, when Jesus was in the wilderness being tempted by the devil, He replaced Satan's lies with the truth found in God's Word. He replied saying, "It is written," and then filled in the blank. Even when Satan twisted Scripture by quoting it out of context, Jesus knowledgably refuted the lie with the truth of that passage.

Paul wrote to Timothy, urging him to "study to show [himself] approved unto God…rightly dividing the word of truth" (2 Tim. 2:15, KJV). Without studying, memorizing, and meditating upon the "word of truth," we have no weapon with which to fight against not just a good liar but the father of all lies. All of us know that in order to do well on a test, much study and memorization are required. Why should it be any different when facing trials and tests in life? We are to use our knowledge of Scripture to fight back, just as Jesus did.

Faith Fact: In a recent Gallup survey, only two out of ten people could identify who delivered the Sermon on the Mount.[6]

While technology can certainly be a deterrent to our spiritual lives with its ceaseless distractions, it can also be a wonderfully useful aid in helping us "download" truth into our hearts and minds. Here are a few examples of what you can do to bulk up your truth belt:

- Download sermons and worship music onto your iPod or MP3 player
- Search the Internet to find podcasts of excellent Bible teachers
- Install an application on your smart phone that supplies Scriptures at your fingertips
- Record sermons and watch them at night before bedtime instead of the latest reality show
- Sign up on a ministry's website to have mini sermons, articles, and verses of the day sent to your in-box
- Listen to a Christian radio station

As beneficial as listening to sermons and teachings can be, it is vitally important that you spend time in God's Word by yourself. Turn off the TV, put your cell phone on silent, and give your undivided attention to the Bible and its Author. Ask Him to be your teacher. Our Knight has gone up to His heavenly kingdom for a little while, but He gave us His Spirit to "teach [us] all things" and "guide [us] into all truth" until He comes back for us (John 14:26; 16:13).

THE BREASTPLATE OF RIGHTEOUSNESS

One of *Merriam-Webster's* definitions for *righteousness* is "acting in accord with divine or moral law: free from guilt or sin."[7] Without the work of Christ, man was powerless to become right with God. Praise Jesus for His redeeming sacrifice! Christ died not only to take away our sins but also to give us His righteousness. The moment we accepted Him as our Lord and Savior, we were immediately imbued with His righteousness. Paul tells us in Philippians that we don't have our own righteousness, as those under the old covenant strove to attain; we have "that [righteousness] which is through faith in Christ" (Phil. 3:9).

Subsequent to girding ourselves with truth, strapping on our breastplate of righteousness is of utmost importance. This piece of armor is the assurance of our right standing before God. Many Christians today carry a burden of condemnation, one that weighs them down with feelings of guilt, shame, and unworthiness. They feel they've failed God in some way and therefore He's no longer interested in blessing, using, or even protecting them. This is another successful strategy of Satan. If he can get us to feel unworthy and unrighteous in the eyes of God, he can effectively cripple our Christian walk and cause us to crumble into mush on the battlefront. We must know that the Prince of the kingdom for which we fight sees us as righteous!

None of us were saved based on our merits. There was no talent, no amount of money, no altruistic deed, no pious prayer that could ever earn our salvation. We were accepted into God's kingdom on the grounds of Christ's righteousness, which He gives to every believer, and we still stand before God based on that life-changing truth. Whenever the devil whispers into your ear that you crossed the line, that you're useless, that you've backslid way too far this time, you can know without a doubt that God sees you through His perfect Son, Jesus Christ. He sees a righteous person!

The apostle Paul is a tremendous example of a man who wore this breastplate well. Before he was converted on the road to Damascus, Paul, then named Saul, was a chief persecutor of Christians. He encouraged the violent stoning of Stephen, the first Christian martyr, and "[breathed] out murderous threats" against God's disciples, arrested them, and threw them into jail (Acts 9:2). Early on, many Christians even disbelieved Paul had experienced a true conversion and continued to fear him! Some members of the early church said his "bodily presence [was] weak" and that his speech was "contemptible" (2 Cor. 10:10, KJV).

If his background doesn't scream, "Grounds for discouragement!" I don't know whose does. Paul had *puh-lenty* of good excuses to throw in the towel and leave all the beatings, shipwrecks, and prison cells behind for a nice hacienda on a Judean hillside. But instead of giving into a feeling of uselessness and unworthiness, Paul said this:

> But by the grace of God I am what I am: and his grace which was bestowed upon me was not in vain; but I laboured more abundantly than they all: yet not I, but the grace of God which was with me.
> —1 CORINTHIANS 15:10, KJV

This is a brilliant, close-up look at Paul's breastplate. It didn't matter how wicked he'd been. It didn't matter if other believers thought him to be a charlatan out to imprison or kill them. It didn't matter what he looked like or how well he spoke. All that mattered was that he was standing on Christ's righteousness alone.

Many in the body of Christ are happy to accept their righteous position before God, but they do little if anything to act like they hold that precious position. In other words, they're content to go through the motions of Christianity: attending church, singing the songs, saying amen at the proper times, participating in a weekly Bible study, and giving thanks before meals. They're satisfied to talk the talk, but when it comes to walking the walk, they say they're "righteous before God, and it doesn't matter what man thinks." Of course, this is partly true; it doesn't matter what man thinks. However, our breastplate symbolizes more than just our righteousness of Christ. It symbolizes the righteousness of Christians.

Ephesians 4:23–24 says we are "to be made new in the attitude of your minds; and to put on the new self, created to be like God in true righteousness and holiness." God doesn't swoop down from heaven and put on our new self for us. While our names are written in the Lamb's Book of Life in heaven, we have an active role in living the Christian life on this earth (Rev. 3:5). If we don't live according to the Word of God and instead frolic about the battlefield like Bambi through a meadow, we'll become easy targets for the best of sharpshooters. We can't complain when we're hit, because we were never prepared to fight in the first place.

Also, if we aren't living righteously on Earth, how effective can our testimonies be to others? Many unbelievers today aren't being saved because they don't see a difference between their lifestyles and the lifestyles of Christians they know. James 4:4 says that to be friends with the world is to be an enemy of God. Remember back to chapter 2: we are to be salt and light in the world.

I have been one of those body parts of Christ who was simply a "pew-warmer," sitting on the sidelines of the greatest game in the universe. In the midst of my eating disorder and prior to it, I harbored pride, practiced a modern-day form of idolatry, and turned to the world for its medical remedies instead of to the Great Physician Himself. I felt unworthy to talk about Jesus with others because my own life failed to reflect Him. I didn't feel I could be victorious over temptations to overexercise or undereat because every time I tried, the enemy made me feel defenseless and defeated. After I repented before the Lord and put on the breastplate of righteousness, I was confident, protected, ready for battle, and excited to share Christ again. What incredible empowerment comes from understanding and accepting our right standing before God!

THE SHOES OF PEACE

Ah, shoes. Bright-colored tennis shoes, rhinestone-studded flip-flops, summery espadrilles, sizzling stilettos. Every occasion, from going for a jog to going to a wedding, calls for a special pair of shoes. If we were going to a reenactment of an ancient Roman battle, that too would call for a unique breed of shoe designed solely—no pun intended—for the purpose of stabilizing a soldier on the battlefield.

In Paul's day, Roman soldiers wore *caligae*, a sort of military boot that looked more like sandals. These boots were made of thick leather and were ventilated on the upper part with hobnails protecting the soles. These hobnails lent themselves to the soldiers' surefootedness in battle, even on slick ground and precarious inclines.[8]

Faith Fact: Scholars suggest that the reason many Roman sculptures of soldiers are barefoot is because the boots were painted on.[9]

There's a logical explanation as to why these military shoes come third in the arming process. First, we put on the belt of truth because Jesus is truth personified, and without Him, we have no foundation from which to build and no defense against the lies of Satan. Second, we put on the breastplate of righteousness, which means living according to the truth of Christ. Righteousness, then, leads us to peace. We no longer wonder where we stand with God, and we no longer struggle to prove our worth to Him because He is our righteousness. In a battle that's being waged against our mind and emotions, it's essential that we arm ourselves with the inner peace only God can give.

In today's shaky political, economical, and social climate, Americans are searching for peace, security, and the formula for how to truly be happy. People turn to self-help books, spiritual gurus, yoga and meditation, prescription drugs, and even Oprah to obtain some semblance of peace. Listen, sister, if you've been searching for tranquility and a respite for your soul, look no further than your Savior. Ephesians 2:14 tells us, "He himself is our peace"! If we can lay a hold of that truth, we can go victoriously into battle neither shaken nor afraid.

Franklin D. Roosevelt's "fireside chats" during the Great Depression and Churchill's inspirational messages during World War II brought immense hope to America and Britain when morale was at its lowest. As they were the voices families daily tuned in to hear in the midst of uncertainty, Jesus Christ should be the voice from whom we receive our peace. He is there in the "airwaves," ready to encourage us when the prognosis is grim, when the future looks bleak, when the battle rages relentlessly. All we have to do is tune in to Him. The peace He gives is the foundation we stand on during battle, just as *caligae* are what the Romans stood on as they conquered.

How are we to go into this worry-ridden world and preach the gospel (the Good News) if our own heart is ill at ease and our mind is filled with angst? Jesus prophesied that in the Last Days there would be great distress in the land and that men's hearts would fail them because of fear (Luke 21:23, 26). If God's people are without peace in such troubling times as these, our hearts will fail alongside those of unbelievers and our testimonies will be rendered powerless.

Jesus also told us we are not to worry about what we eat, drink, or wear. If we seek His kingdom first, He said, all those practical things will be given to us (Matt. 6:31, 33). We can worry until the cows come home, but that won't change one thing. In fact, the only thing it's guaranteed to do is make us unproductive.

Without the shoes of the gospel of peace, we sadly choose to go through life fending for ourselves, fighting battles Jesus longs to help us win.

Galatians 5 counts peace as one of the nine fruit of the Spirit. It stands to reason that we cannot have true peace without the Holy Spirit. After my dad passed away (just seven months ago at the time of this writing), many people approached my mom, brother, and me to say, "You all seem so strong," and, "It's incredible how at peace you are." At the funeral, the three of us had stood at the front of the auditorium and each reflected on the finest man we'd ever known. There is no natural explanation for how we were able to stand and speak at the funeral without our words dissolving into mournful gasps and without our eyes flooding with the tears that hovered just beneath the surface. There is no natural explanation for how, in the midst of our grief and heartache, there was a sense of calm and a sensation of peace that enveloped us just as the branches of an oak tree shield the worn and weary from the wrath of the noonday sun. The supernatural explanation is found in this precious fruit of peace.

Isaiah 26:3 says God will "keep him in perfect peace, whose mind is stayed on [God]" (NKJV). Jesus told us, "Let not your heart be troubled. Trust in God" (John 14:1). As we put our faith in Christ, trusting Him completely, and meditate on the promises of His unchanging Word, we will have stillness within our souls, even as the world spins into chaos around us.

Even as Jesus went to Golgotha to receive the most excruciating form of torture ever devised by mankind, He carried a calmness and resolve that came from the perfect peace He possessed. Christ told us that in order to be His follower, we are to pick up our crosses every day and follow Him (Luke 9:23). We'd better make sure we have on the proper shoes for such a journey.

Faith Fact: The word *excruciating* comes from the Latin word *excruciatus*, meaning "out of the cross."[10]

THE SHIELD OF FAITH

This one's a biggie. Paul says that "above all" we are to put on the shield of faith (Eph. 6:16, KJV). Shields were the most important piece of an ancient soldier's armor. The Roman shield, called a *scutum*, wasn't some flimsy, Frisbee-like apparatus that was merely for show. On the contrary, the *scutum* was four feet long and two and a half feet wide—the size of a really chubby eight-year-old. This thing guarded the soldier's whole body! It was slightly curved, which not only better absorbed heavy blows but could deflect arrows altogether.[11]

Paul says that with this shield, we can "quench the fiery darts of the wicked" (Eph. 6:16, KJV). These Roman shields were doubly useful, because they were lined with metal. When the enemy would rain fiery arrows upon the opposing army, all the soldiers had to do was hurl their shields over their heads, making a fireproof roof for themselves. (If you want to get a visual of this, check out my favorite movie, *Gladiator*.) The Roman army actually had a formation called the tortoise, in which their risen shields resembled a turtle's shell.

Fiery arrows are a very apt analogy to describe Satan's attacks. They are swift and silent, like a venomous cobra in high grass, able to catch a soldier off guard. On top of that, the Roman arrows were sometimes tipped with poison, so even if the initial impact didn't kill the soldier, the toxin seeping into his veins eventually would. Just like fiery or poisonous darts, an attack from Satan, if not defended against, can inject a bitter dose of despair, depression, and discouragement into our minds and leave a lingering sting wherever it touches.

Without our shield, we leave any empty spots between our armor open for attack. First Kings records King Ahab's death, which happened this way:

> But someone drew his bow at random and hit the king of Israel between the sections of his armor. The king told his chariot driver, "Wheel around and get me out of the fighting. I've been wounded." All day long the battle raged, and the king was propped up in his chariot facing the Arameans. The blood from his wound ran onto the floor of the chariot, and that evening he died.
>
> —1 Kings 22:34–35

Satan's soldiers are assigned to study our weaknesses and stalk us like lions, looking for an opportunity to shoot one of their darts between the empty places of our armor (1 Pet. 5:8). It's no wonder the Bible tells us to put the shield on "above all." We are commanded to defend ourselves against such insidiously destructive assaults.

In all of history, beginning in the Garden of Eden, the first item on Satan's agenda has been to create doubt. He was able to deceive Eve into questioning God and has been trapping mankind with the snare of doubt ever since. When we say we have faith in someone, we mean we believe they'll do what they've said. We find them trustworthy and reliable. For example, last year I had nasal surgery for my deviated septum. I didn't fear I wouldn't wake up from the anesthesia, and I wasn't afraid I'd end up with a nose that belonged on Mount Rushmore. I had faith in my surgeon, and I knew I was in good hands—or at least I knew my nose was. This is the sort of faith we are to have in God.

Hebrews 11:1 defines faith as being "the substance of things hoped for, the evidence of things not seen" (KJV). The rest of the chapter, popularly called the "Hall of Faith," chronicles Old Testament figures who serve as inspiring examples of people who lived by faith. Take Noah. Noah lived in a world that had never seen rain, and yet he was told by God to build a floating zoo that would preserve him, his family, and the lucky critters from the impending floodwaters. Noah obeyed the Lord, and for one hundred years he cut timber and shaped, transported, and erected the massive beams required to construct the world's first cruise ship.

You can imagine the ridicule he must've received. "Noah, you've lost your mind! You believe God told you to build a what? What's a boat? A drop of water has never fallen from heaven, and you're telling us you're building a boat to survive some silly sky-water?" We can be sure Satan tried to cause a mental flood of doubt to wash away Noah's faith in God's command. But with his shield of faith, Noah and his loved ones escaped God's wrath unscathed on board their personal ocean liner.

Faith Fact: The evidence for the Genesis flood is all around us. The features of our planet proclaim its catastrophic past, from the sea beds to the Grand Canyon. Encased in layers of sedimentary rock miles within the earth's crust are billions of dead plants and animals that were buried very quickly.[12]

All throughout the Bible we read of men and women being called to do things that seemed preposterous to secular eyes. But as long as they held fast to their faith in God, they could face the sneers of scoffers and the darts of Satan and have victory. When writing to young Timothy, Paul exhorts the young man to "fight the good fight of faith" (1 Tim. 6:12, KJV). It's not a fight without faith!

I can think of no other place in America wherein young people's faith is challenged and attacked more than secular colleges and universities. More and more professors and university curricula seek to dissolve the believability of one's faith by presenting intellectual theories, such as evolution, as superior to "arcane" or "mythological" biblical truths. In an age of religious pluralism, God is viewed as more of an impersonal force than an almighty, transcendent Person. These academic "realists" don't recognize the concept of God because, they say, He is not observable (evolution has never been observed, might I add). Furthermore, objective, biblical notions such as moral guilt don't fit in an ethically fragmented framework of relativism. In other words, what's right to you is right.

Outside the walls of these indoctrinating institutions, college students are surrounded by pleasure-seeking peers who are experimenting with all kinds of harmful, self-satisfying practices in their searches to find themselves. From drugs and alcohol to profanity and sexual promiscuity, the college atmosphere is one of the devil's most beloved playgrounds. It is in this fertile soil, rife with the impressionable minds of young people and the vim and vigor of their quest for knowledge of all kinds, that the enemy can plant weeds of cynicism and disbelief and sow seeds of discord between students and the mentors whose godly wisdom they once respected.

Faith Fact: A recent UCLA study found that 52 percent of the students said they attended religious services frequently the year before entering college, but their attendance had dropped to 29 percent by their junior year.[13]

God doesn't give college students a big box of faith as a high school graduation present, nor does He fortify our cereal with it each morning in the real world. The only way to wield faith like a weapon is to familiarize ourselves with the truth of God's Word. By knowing the truth, we can successfully defend our beliefs, fight the fires of doubt, and even reinforce the faith of those around us while sharing an instigating spark of the gospel with cynics and unbelievers.

Building our faith is a lot like working out! I'm serious! We can't strengthen our muscles by lounging on the La-Z-Boy watching exercise DVDs, and we don't develop spiritual strength merely by knowing theological terms or reading Christian books. James, the brother of Jesus, wrote that faith without works is dead (James 2:17). Listen to the Lord, and if you hear Him telling you to do something, be faithful and do it to it! You may not be able to visualize the results, and people might tell you you're taking a risk or being unrealistic, but remind yourself that faith means placing your confidence in God, not in your own abilities or those of anyone else. Remember:

> Now faith is the substance of things hoped for, the evidence of things not seen. For by it the elders obtained a good testimony. By faith we understand that the worlds were framed by the word of God, so that the things which are seen were not made of things which are visible.
>
> —HEBREWS 11:1–3, NKJV

Faith Fact: Martin Luther King Jr. said, "Faith is taking the first step even when you don't see the whole staircase."[14]

THE HELMET OF SALVATION

Everyone who's ever learned to ride a bike is familiar with helmets. I distinctly remember complaining every time my riding instructor handed me my less-than-stylish helmet before I got on my first horse, Buttercup. I was only four years old, but I was not a fan of helmet hair.

Helmets are indispensable pieces of protective gear in numerous occupations and pastimes today, from construction and firefighting to football and rock climbing. Secondary to the shield, helmets were the most important piece of ancient soldiers' armor, and they're still worn by troops today to protect them from bullets and shell fragments. Whether a young equestrian as I once was or a soldier defending his nation, an individual can sustain various bodily injuries such as a dislocated shoulder, a fractured ankle, or even a broken back, but head wounds can often result in prolonged or irreversible brain damage, if not instant death. Without the helmet of salvation, we put ourselves at extreme risk for a satanic assault within our own ears.

Fit Fact: Helmet use has been estimated to reduce the risk of head injury by 85 percent.[15]

In 1 Thessalonians, Paul calls this helmet the "hope of salvation" (1 Thess. 5:8, NKJV). We use the word *hope* rather flippantly today: "I hope it's sunny this weekend," or, "I really hope I get the job!" However, in a biblical context, hope is something much more powerful. In his letter to Titus, Paul said that "faith and knowledge [rest] on the hope of eternal life" (Titus 1:2). If faith and knowledge are to "rest" upon hope, it would certainly behoove us to guard it!

A helmet is needed to protect our hope, because hope is very much a matter of the mind. It is something we ponder, understand, and even look forward to (Titus 2:13). The picture of protective headgear reminds us that we are to have the "mind of Christ," full of His plans, thoughts, truth, and purposes (1 Cor. 2:16). Having the mind of our Lord goes far beyond simply having an intellectual knowledge of the salvation we've been given. We are to spiritually equip ourselves with the wisdom of God, personified in Jesus Christ (1 Cor. 1:24). It is through this wisdom that we can stand victorious against a barrage of demonic darts and oppressive affronts.

Christians throughout history have faced unthinkable persecution and harassment on account of their faith. Even in our own nation, we are beginning to see a spirit of antichrist trying to silence us from proclaiming the Good News of Jesus. Today's intelligentsia, composed of our political leaders and university professors, seek to make us question and reject the very One who gave His life to save us. When we face attacks, threats, or hurtful ostracism from friends, coworkers, and even the government, or when doubts begin to creep into our thoughts as anti-Christian ideologies are propagated, it is the hope of the finished work of Jesus that is our anchor of confidence against all fear and uncertainty.

Faith Fact: In 2009, the Democrat speaker of the Pennsylvania House banned prayers prayed in Jesus's name before the state legislature.[16]

To gain God's wisdom, the mind of Christ, we must spend time with Him in His Word. As a college freshman, I let my devotional time dwindle until it consisted of a mere five to ten minutes of arbitrary verse selection and slapdash note-taking at night. My Bible went from being my rock to a bedside table. I reasoned I was too tired, too busy, too distracted to spend adequate time reading God's Word, and my helmet began to slip. I became easily discouraged, overly sensitive, and felt self-pitying as other girls in the dorm went out partying, meeting cute guys, staying out late, seemingly have the time of their lives. *I should be having fun with them. I'm eighteen years old. If I don't live it up now, when will I?*

I'd allowed the hope of my salvation to become the hindrance to a worldly lifestyle. The wisdom of God had been replaced with the foolishness of college kids. If Satan owned a business, it would be called C & C Towing. He specializes in *corrupting* and *confusing* the minds of believers so he can then tow them across town to his impound lot, where they no longer pose a threat to his kingdom. If our minds are full of confusion and ungodly thoughts, we can't think on God's purposes for us, and as a result, we stray from His path and miss out on His plans.

Jesus gave us incredible encouragement when it comes to operating with the helmet of salvation. In Matthew 10, He prophesied that the apostles would be "brought before governors and kings for My sake, as a testimony to them and to the Gentiles. But when they deliver you up, do not worry about how or what you should speak. For it will be given to you in that hour what you should speak" (Matt. 10:18–20, NKJV). It's guaranteed that there will be times when we'll be met with hostility because of what we believe. In such instances, all we need do is trust God because our minds are "of Christ"! God's own wisdom will pour forth from our lips.

In the New Testament, the apostles' accusers often marveled at the men's authoritative speech. Peter, an uneducated fisherman, spoke so well and with such authority that the only way the Sanhedrin knew to deal with him was to plot to kill him (Acts 5:33). The power of God in these accounts and in every believer's life enables us to communicate beyond our natural talents or ability. As Christians, we mustn't run from confrontation or bury our heads in the sand when opposition approaches. Peter, inspired by the Holy Spirit, instructed us to "always be prepared to give an answer to everyone who asks you to give the reason for the hope that you have" (1 Pet. 3:15). Jesus has promised to supply us with the words to say, but we can only do so if we make His thoughts our thoughts by knowing His Word.

THE SWORD OF THE SPIRIT

Time to get offensive—but in a good way. While the other five pieces of our armor defend us, the sword of the Spirit is the mighty, all-sufficient weapon with which we drive the enemy back, resisting him, preventing him from stalking us like a sniper as he waits for one of our defenses to collapse. Ephesians 6:17 tells us this sword is the "word of God."

So we fully understand how we're to fight with words, let's look at two forms of the term *word* used in the New Testament. First off, there's the Greek word *logos*, which refers to a spoken word that expresses the thoughts and intents of the speaker. It has to do with the logic of what's being communicated. The first chapter of John's Gospel uses *logos* when it speaks of Christ as the Word. In Ephesians 6, however, the Greek word used is *rhema*, which means a "thing spoken; a word or saying of any kind" that doesn't require logic to be understood, but rather belief.[17]

Romans 10:17 uses *rhema*, saying, "Faith cometh by hearing, and hearing by the word [*rhema*] of God" (KJV). We were saved not while hearing a Socratic debate or the philosophizing of erudite theological experts. Our faith came free of a crash course in systematic theology or a seminary degree. We were saved simply by believing the *rhema* words concerning Christ that were spoken or shown to us in Scripture. That is how *rhema* words continue to operate in the lives of believers. Jesus said, "The Spirit gives life; the flesh counts for nothing. The words I have spoken to you are spirit and they are life" (John 6:63). The "words" He spoke of are *rhema* words that become personal revelations and living sayings as we read the Scriptures. If you've ever felt the all-encompassing joy and awe of reading a passage of the Bible that all but jumped off the page to give you a hug, wipe away your tears, or speak much-needed encouragement, you've felt the power of God's *rhema*.

There is nothing more powerful than the Word of God in a Christian's life. Hebrews 4:12 describes the Word of God as "living and active, and sharper than any two-edged sword, piercing even to the division of soul and spirit, and of joints and marrow, and is a discerner of the thoughts and intents of the heart" (NKJV). Allow me to sum it up: the sword we carry beats the pants off Luke Skywalker's dinky lightsaber. And not only is it alive, but it is sharper and even more supernatural than Excalibur. The legends may hold that the enchanted sword penetrated a stone, but did King Arthur ever pierce through people's spirits with it?

Metal swords wielded by men affect only the external frame of their enemies—their flesh. However, the sword of the Spirit cuts to the core of men's souls. For example, on the Day of Pentecost, ten days after Christ's ascension into heaven, Peter's preaching "cut to the heart" of the listeners, compelling them to ask, "Brothers, what shall we do?" (Acts 2:37). Peter, speaking by the power of the Spirit, had so gripped the hearts of those gathered, piercing them with the sword of God's Word, that they were practically chomping at the bit to find out how to make Jesus Lord of their lives!

I'm sure most of us have heard at least one sermon similar to that one, one that seemed to call our name, saying, "This is just for you!" Next time you're sitting at church hearing God's Word and it feels as if it's just you and the Lord alone in the sanctuary, or when you're holding the Psalms open in your lap and the poetry materializes into guidance for your present circumstance, take heart: you've just been pierced with the sword of the Spirit!

Jesus displayed His mastery of the sword while in the wilderness being tempted by Satan. Satan approached Jesus with the three predominant temptations he's used throughout history, what John characterized as the "lust of the flesh, the lust of the eyes, and the pride of life" (1 John 2:16, KJV). According to biblical scholar Adam Clarke, "the lust of the flesh" implies "sensual and impure desires which seek their gratification in women, strong drink, delicious [foods], and the like." "The lust of the eyes" refers to "inordinate desires after finery of every kind, gaudy dress, splendid houses, superb furniture, expensive equipage, trappings, and decorations of all sorts." The "pride of life" implicates "hunting after honors, titles, and pedigrees; boasting of ancestry, family connections, great offices, and honorable acquaintance."[18]

Right off the bat Satan sought to tempt Jesus's flesh. It had been at least forty days since Jesus's last meal. (I don't know about you, but my tummy starts rumbling after three hours, let alone forty days!) Satan said, "If you are the Son of God, command these stones become bread." Had Jesus succumbed to the temptation to, in His divinity, turn a pile of rocks into a sirloin steak, Satan would have destroyed His mission by getting Jesus to act outside the will of His Father. Jesus said He came "not to be served...but to give His life as a ransom for many" (Matt. 20:28). Never did He perform a miracle for Himself.

So what did Jesus do? He pulled out a sword, stating, "It is written, 'Man shall not live by bread alone, but by every word that proceeds from the mouth of God'" (Matt. 4:4, NKJV; see also Deut. 8:3). Jesus would indeed receive nourishment, but it wouldn't be derived from natural food. Satan, unable to appeal to Jesus's flesh due to the fearsome blow of the sword, moved on to the lust of the eyes.

In temptation number two, Satan, "took Him up into the holy city, set Him on the pinnacle of the temple, and said to Him, 'If You are the Son of God, throw yourself down. For it is written: "He shall give His angels charge over you," and, "In their hands they shall bear you up, lest you dash your foot against a stone"''" (Matt. 4:5–6, NKJV).

Satan upped his game this go-round by quoting Scripture. However, he left out a significant fragment of the Psalm 91 passage: "to keep thee in all your ways" (Ps. 91:11, KJV). This key phrase was shrewdly omitted, because it speaks of provision while we are operating in God's will, not behaving recklessly outside of it.

In the first temptation, Satan tried to tempt Jesus to act independently of His Father. In the second, he tried to get Jesus to act presumptuously by jumping from the heights of the temple, trusting the angels to catch Him. Had Jesus done this, everyone beneath, even the religious rabbis, would've exalted Him, because a tradition held that their Messiah would appear on the temple roof. But Jesus unsheathed another powerful sword, declaring, "It is written again, 'You shall not tempt the LORD your God'" (Matt 4:7, NKJV; see also Deut. 6:16).

We cannot deviate from the will of God and then selfishly demand that He come to our rescue when we're knee-deep in self-made mire. Acting imprudently, living destructively, and then calling on God and His angels to save us is to tempt God, as it vainly misuses such hopeful, promising passages like Psalm 91.

Zero for two, Satan moves on to the pride of life. He takes Jesus from the temple roof to a high mountain and shows Him all the world's kingdoms. He said to Jesus, "All these things I will give You if You will fall down and worship me" (Matt. 4:9, NKJV). Satan was now trying to persuade Jesus to take a shortcut to setting up His messianic kingdom. Knowing the prophecies of how Jesus was to suffer, it was as if Satan were saying, "I can give you an earthly kingdom right here, right now. It's mine to give, and all I require is that you worship me. No need to be forsaken and suffer death!"

The sword chosen next was the final blow:

Away from me, Satan! For it is written: "Worship the Lord your God, and serve him only."

—MATTHEW 4:10

Immediately after that "the devil left Him" (Matt. 4:11). Jesus won! He flawlessly fought the lust of the flesh and eyes and the pride of life by skillfully wielding the sword of the Spirit. By recalling the written word (*logos*) and proclaiming it as spoken power (*rhema*), Jesus resisted a series of great trials, which serves as a shining example of how to appropriate God's Word, brandishing it as an unbeatable weapon against the devil.

Faith Fact: "No temptation has seized you except what is common to man. And God is faithful; he will not let you be tempted beyond what you can bear. But when you are tempted, he will also provide a way out so that you can stand up under it" (1 Cor. 10:13).

FULLY LOADED

Whether fighting unseen forces of evil, fleeing the lures of the flesh, or evading the snares of the world, we must put on the armor to be victorious over every adversary that purposes to push us off God's path through discouragement, deception, complacency, destruction, and seduction.

As the return of Jesus, our Knight on the white horse, draws nearer, the battle on Earth will only intensify. While many may try to convince you that we stand on neutral ground, we'd be wise to remember that Satan is the prince of this world, and we fight on his turf. How can we win if we don't even recognize there's a battle going on? Don't doze off listening to deadly lullabies with verses like, "Live it up! Eat, drink, and be merry! Don't think about tomorrow, live in the moment!"

As Paul said, physical training is of "some value," but "godliness has value for all things" (1 Tim. 4:8). I challenge you to be as disciplined about putting on your armor each morning as you are about eating a healthy breakfast or fitting in your three-mile run before sunup. I urge you to be as devoted to spending time with God each night in prayer and study as you are about seeing your friends at the gym.

I hope and pray that this study of God's armor has helped you understand the vital importance of being prepared, both defensively and offensively, to do battle, not just every once in a while but every day. It should give us great peace and impenetrable confidence to know that we're not untrained, ill-equipped citizens at war. We are disciplined, topnotch soldiers in service to the ultimate

Commanding Officer, who has already conquered all and is coming again to rule and reign!

Faith Fact: "You are from God, little children, and have overcome them; because greater is He who is in you than he who is in the world" (1 John 4:4, NAS).

Appendix A

FOOD FOR YOUR TEMPLE

Sample Meal Plans

Monday	
Breakfast	2 eggs, 1 serving of spelt flake cereal, ¼ cup blueberries, 1 cup nonfat milk, black coffee, 16 oz. water
Snack 1	1 apple with 1 Tbsp. almond butter
Lunch	Turkey sandwich on sprouted bread (such as Ezekiel bread) with veggies, mustard, 1 cup low-fat yogurt, 8 oz. green tea
Snack 2	String cheese, 15 grapes
Dinner	½ cup brown rice, 4 oz. grilled chicken, 1 cup broccoli, 16 oz. water
Optional bedtime snack	1 cup cottage cheese with 1/3 cup pineapple chunks

Tuesday	
Breakfast	Fruit smoothie made with ½ cup low-fat vanilla yogurt, ½ cup nonfat milk, ½ cup frozen blueberries or strawberries, 2 Tbsp. honey, ice (if desired); 16 oz. water
Snack 1	1 banana with 1 Tbsp. natural peanut butter
Lunch	Roast beef sandwich on whole-grain sourdough bread with caramelized onions, ½ cup melon, 8 oz. green tea
Snack 2	Apple slices, 1 oz. cheese
Dinner	4 oz. salmon, 1 cup asparagus, garden salad with 2 Tbsp. low-fat vinaigrette dressing, 16 oz. water
Optional bedtime snack	2 oz. mixed raw nuts (such as almonds, pecans, walnuts), 8 oz. chamomile tea

Wednesday	
Breakfast	1 serving cooked oatmeal with 1 oz. almonds, 1 Tbsp. honey, black coffee, 16 oz. water
Snack 1	4 Tbsp. hummus with 15 baby carrots
Lunch	Chopped pita salad with romaine lettuce, 2 Tbsp. crumbled feta cheese, ½ cup garbanzo beans drained and rinsed, sliced cucumber, 1 chopped whole-wheat pita, 2 Tbsp. low-fat vinaigrette, 8 oz. jasmine tea
Snack 2	2 rice cakes, 1 Tbsp. natural peanut butter
Dinner	4 oz. sirloin steak, 1 medium sweet potato, 1 cup green beans, 16 oz. water
Optional bedtime snack	1 cup low-fat or nonfat vanilla yogurt with 1 Tbsp. honey

Thursday	
Breakfast	Veggie omelet made with 4-6 egg whites; ½ cup strawberries, 16 oz. water, black coffee
Snack 1	Berry smoothie made with 1 cup whole-milk yogurt, 1 cup fresh or frozen berries, 1 Tbsp. unheated honey
Lunch	Tuna salad made with 3-5 oz. water-packed tuna, 2 tsp. omega-3 mayonnaise, chopped onions, peppers, and celery, 1 apple, 8 oz. green tea
Snack 2	1 cup of 2 percent Greek yogurt, 2 tsp. honey
Dinner	4 oz. halibut, ½ cup brown rice, 4 asparagus spears
Optional bedtime snack	½ cup low-fat organic ice cream

	Friday
Breakfast	Veggie frittata made with 1 egg and 5 egg whites, 1 cup broccoli florets, julienned red peppers, chopped onion, 1 Tbsp. extra-virgin olive oil, herbs and sea salt to taste, (Saute vegetables, remove from heat. Then, add olive oil to skillet, and add egg mixture. Spoon the vegetables on top. Cook until set, and flip like a pancake.) 16 oz. water
Snack 1	1 slice sprouted cinnamon-raisin bread (such as Ezekiel 4:9 Bread) with 1 Tbsp. almond butter
Lunch	Salmon salad made with 2 oz. water-packed salmon, 1 Tbsp. omega-3 mayonnaise, chopped onions, peppers, and celery on a bed of romaine lettuce with 2 Tbsp. low-fat vinaigrette dressing, 1 orange, 8 oz. white tea
Snack 2	Organic raw fruit-and-nut bar
Dinner	4 oz. buffalo burger on whole-wheat bun, organic ketchup, ½ cup black beans, unsweetened ice tea or tea sweetened with stevia or xylitol
Optional bedtime snack	1 cup sliced peaches, ½ cup cottage cheese

SERVINGS

When you don't have measuring cups and spoons on hand, just use your eyeballs!

- 4–6 oz: the size of your palm or a deck of cards
- 1 cup of rice or pasta: the size of a tennis ball or ice cream scoop
- 1 cup salad greens: the size of a baseball
- ½ cup cooked veggies: the size of an ice cream scoop
- 1 piece of medium-sized fruit: the size of a tennis ball
- 1 Tbsp. peanut butter: the size of a table tennis ball
- 1 tsp.: the size of a stamp
- 1 cup yogurt: the size of a tennis ball or ice cream scoop
- 1 oz. of cheese: the size of a pair of dice

Appendix B

WORKOUT ROUTINES

*Home Is Where the Health Is—Circuit Training
in Your Living Room*

ROUTINE A

Circuit 1

Exercise	Muscle Groups	Time
Body squat	Glutes, thighs	45 seconds
Triceps dips	Triceps, chest	45 seconds
Crunches	Rectus abdominis (the long muscle of the abdomen, what gives you a "six pack")	45 seconds
Modified push-ups	Chest, triceps, abs	45 seconds
Star jumps	Whole body	45 seconds

Circuit 2

Exercise	Muscle Groups	Time
Knee-to-elbow	Obliques	45 seconds
Burpees	Whole body	45 seconds
Superman	Lower back	45 seconds
Close-arm wall push-ups	Triceps, chest	45 seconds

Circuit 3

Exercise	Muscle Groups	Time
Stationary lunges	Thighs, glutes	45 seconds
Bicycle crunches	Rectus abdominis, obliques	45 seconds
Double punch	Shoulders, upper back	45 seconds
Bridge	Thighs, glutes	45 seconds

Note: Remember to cool down before stretching.

Stretch	Time
Hips/glutes	15–30 seconds each leg
Inner thighs	15–30 seconds
Hamstring	15–30 seconds on each leg
Chest and shoulders	15–30 seconds
Upper back	15–30 seconds
Triceps	15–30 seconds on each arm
Spine twist	15–30 seconds on each side

ROUTINE B

Circuit 1

Exercise	Equipment Needed	Muscle Groups	Time
Lateral lunge with shoulder press	Pair of light-weight dumbbells	Glutes, thighs, shoulders	45 seconds
Chest flies	Pair of dumbbells, exercise ball	Chest, core, hamstrings, glutes	45 seconds
Bent-over row	Pair of dumbbells	Upper back, biceps	45 seconds
Triceps extension	Light resistance band	Triceps	45 seconds

Circuit 2

Exercise	Equipment Needed	Muscle Groups	Time
Plié squat with bicep curl	Pair of medium-weight dumbbells	Glutes, inner and outer thighs, biceps	45 seconds
Dumbbell chest press	Pair of medium-weight dumbbells, exercise ball	Chest, core, hamstrings	45 seconds

Exercise	Equipment Needed	Muscle Groups	Time
Reverse flies	Light-weight dumbbells, exercise ball	Upper and lower back, hamstrings	45 seconds
Ball pass	Exercise ball	Lower abdominals	45 seconds

Circuit 3

Exercise	Equipment Needed	Muscle Groups	Time
Alternating lunges with oblique twist	One heavy dumbbell	Thighs, glutes, hamstrings, obliques	45 seconds
Decline push-ups	Exercise ball	Chest, triceps, abs	45 seconds
Biceps curls	Medium resistance band	Biceps	45 seconds
Exercise ball crunch	Exercise ball	Rectus abdominis	45 seconds

Note: Remember to cool down as you did in Routine A.

Stretch	Time
Quad stretch	15–30 on seconds each leg
One-arm chest stretch	15–30 seconds
Hamstring stretch	15–30 on seconds each leg
Back extension	15–30 seconds
Upper back	15–30 seconds
Triceps	15–30 on seconds each arm
Spine twist	15–30 on seconds each side

ROUTINE C

Circuit 1

Exercise	Equipment Needed	Muscle Groups	Reps
Military press	Pair of light-weight dumbbells, exercise ball	Shoulders, core	15–20
Dumbbell pull-over	One heavy dumbbell, exercise ball	Chest, back, triceps, core, glutes, hamstrings	12–15
Incline chest press	Medium pair of dumbbells, exercise ball	Chest, core	12–15
Single arm lat pull-down	Medium resistance band	Back, biceps	12–15 each side

Circuit 2

Exercise	Equipment Needed	Muscle Groups	Reps
Dumbbell push-ups with alternating row	Pair of dumbbells (any weight)	Chest, shoulders, back, core	12 push-ups
One-arm rear delt fly	Medium resistance band	Back, shoulders	12–15 on each side
Headbangers	Pair of light-weight dumbbells, exercise ball	Triceps, core	12–15
Ball roll-out	Exercise ball	Abs, back	10–12

Circuit 3

Exercise	Equipment Needed	Muscle Groups	Reps
Triceps kickback	Pair of light dumbbells, exercise ball	Triceps, core	12–15

Exercise	Equipment Needed	Muscle Groups	Reps
Hammer curls	Medium resistance band	Biceps	12–15
Upright row	Medium pair of dumbbells	Shoulders	12–15
Ball side-to-side	Exercise ball	Obliques	6–8 each side

Note: Remember to cool down.

Stretch	Time
Kneeling chest stretch	15–30 seconds on each arm
Supine shoulder stretch	15–30 seconds
Bent-over shoulder stretch	15–30 seconds on each arm
Bent-over shoulder flexion stretch	15–30 seconds
Core stretch	15–30 seconds
Triceps	15–30 seconds on each arm
Spine twist	15–30 seconds on each side

ROUTINE D

Circuit 1

Exercise	Equipment Needed	Muscle Groups	Reps
Lunge on the ball	One heavy dumbbell, exercise ball	Glutes, thighs	12–15 on each leg
Ball roll-ins	Exercise ball	Hamstrings	12–15
Plié squat with heel raise	One heavy dumbbell	Glutes, inner and outer thighs, calves	12–15
Butt blaster	Medium resistance band	Glutes	12–15 on each side

Circuit 2

Exercise	Equipment Needed	Muscle Groups	Reps
Squat	Medium resistance band	Glutes, thighs	12–15
Ball calf raise	Exercise ball, medium pair of dumbbells	Calves	15–20
Curtsy lunge	Self	Glutes, thighs	12–15 on each side
Stiff leg dead-lift	Pair of medium dumbbells	Hamstrings, lower back	12–15

Circuit 3

Exercise	Equipment Needed	Muscle Groups	Time
Bridge on the ball	Exercise ball	Glutes, hamstrings	12–15
Ball lift	Exercise ball	Inner and outer thighs	10–12 on each side
Squat with leg extension	Wall, exercise ball	Glutes, thighs	10–12 on each side
Seated calf raise	Chair, heavy pair of dumbbells	Calves	15–20

Note: Remember to cool down.

Stretch	Time
Lunge stretch	15–30 seconds
Bent-over inner thigh stretch	15–30 seconds on each side
Hips/glutes	15–30 seconds on each side
Inner thigh	15–30 seconds
Hamstrings	15–30 seconds on each side
Calf	15–30 each side
Spine twist	15–30 seconds on each side

Time to Hit the Club! Circuit Training at the Gym: Routine A

Circuit 1

Exercise	Muscle Groups	Time
Smith machine squat	Glutes, thighs	45 seconds
Chest press machine	Chest, triceps	45 seconds
Leg extension machine	Thighs	45 seconds
Cable row	Back, biceps	45 seconds

Circuit 2

Exercise	Muscle Groups	Time
Incline leg press	Glutes, thighs	45 seconds
Decline bench press	Chest, triceps	45 seconds
Lying hamstring curl	Hamstrings	45 seconds
Roman chair knee-lift	Lower abs	45 seconds

Circuit 3

Exercise	Muscle Groups	Time
BOSU squat jump	Thighs, glutes, abs	45 seconds
Cable flies	Chest	45 seconds
Wide grip lat pull-downs	Back, shoulders, biceps	45 seconds
Military press	Shoulders	45 seconds

Note: Remember to cool down before stretching.

Stretch	Time
Hips/glutes	15–30 seconds on each leg
Inner thigh	15–30 seconds
Hamstring	15–30 seconds on each leg
Chest and shoulders	15–30 seconds
Upper back	15–30 seconds
Triceps	15–30 seconds on each arm

Stretch	Time
Spine twist	15–30 seconds on each side

Routine B

Circuit 1

Exercise	Muscle Groups	Time
Barbell bench press	Chest, triceps	45 seconds
Assisted wide-grip pull-ups	Back	45 seconds
Cable curls	Biceps	45 seconds
BOSU side plank	Obliques	20 seconds each side

Circuit 2

Exercise	Muscle Groups	Time
Incline dumbbell fly	Chest	45 seconds
Dumbbell row	Back, biceps	45 seconds
Cable overhead triceps extension	Triceps	45 seconds
Decline sit-up with medicine ball	Upper abs	45 seconds

Circuit 3

Exercise	Muscle Groups	Time
BOSU push-up	Chest, triceps	45 seconds
Rear-delt fly on machine	Upper back	45 seconds
Assisted triceps dip	Triceps	45 seconds
Preacher curls	Biceps	45 seconds

Note: Remember to cool down before stretching.

Stretch	Time
Kneeling chest stretch	15–30 seconds on each arm
Supine shoulder stretch	15–30 seconds

Stretch	Time
Bent-over shoulder stretch	15–30 seconds on each arm
Bent-over shoulder flexion stretch	15–30 seconds
Core stretch	15–30 seconds
Triceps	15–30 seconds on each arm
Spine twist	15–30 seconds on each side

ROUTINE C

Circuit 1

Exercise	Muscle Groups	Time
BOSU side lunge	Glutes, thighs	Approx. 22 seconds on each leg
Dumbbell step-up	Glutes, thighs	45 seconds
Smith machine plié squat	Inner thighs	45 seconds
Standing calf raise machine	Calves	45 seconds

Circuit 2

Exercise	Muscle Groups	Time
Leg press	Thighs	45 seconds
BOSU stiff leg dead-lift	Hamstrings, lower back	45 seconds
One-legged squat with cable	Glutes, thighs	Approx. 22 seconds on each leg
Calf raises on incline leg press	Calves	45 seconds

Circuit 3

Exercise	Muscle Groups	Time
Hack squat machine	Thighs, glutes, abs	45 seconds
Seated hamstring curl	Hamstrings	45 seconds
BOSU lunge	Glutes, thighs	45 seconds
Seated calf raise machine	Calves	45 seconds

Note: Remember to cool down.

Stretch	Time
Lunge stretch	15–30 seconds
Bent-over inner thigh stretch	15–30 seconds on each side
Hips/glutes	15–30 seconds on each side
Inner thighs	15–30 seconds
Hamstrings	15–30 seconds on each side
Calf	15–30 each side
Spine twist	15–30 seconds on each side

OPTIONAL EXERCISES FOR PARTNERS

Exercise	Muscle Groups	Time
Ball toss	Rectus abdominis (the six-pack muscle)	45 seconds
Exercise ball push	Obliques	45 seconds
V's	Shoulders, upper back	45 seconds
BOSU toss	Obliques	Approx. 22 seconds on each side
Mid-row	Back, glutes, thighs	45 seconds
Kneeling twist	Obliques	45 seconds
Squat with chest pass	Glutes, thighs, chest	45 seconds
Floor slams	Shoulders, abs	45 seconds
Lunge with chest pass	Glutes, thighs, chest	45 seconds

NOTES

CHAPTER ONE
MISS UNIVERSITY GRADUATES

1. Rick Warren, The Purpose-Driven Life (Grand Rapids, MI: Zondervan, 2004), 17.

CHAPTER TWO
A TIME TO EVERY PURPOSE

1. Daniel J. DeNoon, "Too Much Salt Hurting Majority of Americans," WebMD, March 26, 2009, http://www.webmd.com/heart/news/20090326/too-much-salt-hurting-two-thirds-of-americans (accessed November 16, 2009).

2. Ralph Waldo Emerson, quoted at Quoteland.com, http://www.quoteland. com/topic/Light-Quotes/539/ (accessed May 21, 2011).

3. BibleGateway.com

4. Strong's Greek Lexicon, available at Eliyah.com, http://www.eliyah.com/cgi-bin/strongs.cgi?file=greeklexicon&index=walk (accessed April 1, 2010).

5. "Sedentary Lifestyle Accelerates Again," The Washington Post, January 28, 2008, http://www.washingtonpost.com/wp-dyn/content/article/2008/01/28/AR2008012802081.html, (accessed December 22, 2009).

6. Bible Study Tools, "Tekton," BibleStudyTools.com, Greek source- biblestudy-tools.com/lexicons/greek/kjv/tekton.html (accessed June 7, 2011).

7. Council for Secular Humanism, www.secularhumanism.com (accessed January 13, 2010).

8. Greg Epstein, quoted in Human Chaplaincy at Harvard, http://harvard-humanist.org/index.php?option=com_content&view=article&id=7&ltemid=2 (accessed January 13, 2010).

CHAPTER THREE
CHEZ YAHWEH: WHAT WOULD GOD'S RESTAURANT BE COOKIN'?

1. The Waltham Clinic, "Weight Loss," http://thewalthamclinic.com/weight_loss.html (accessed June 7, 2011).

2. Hayim H. Donin, To Be A Jew: A Guide To Jewish Observance In Contemporary Life (New York: Basic Books, 1991), 99.

3. Amazing Health, "Unclean Animals," http://amazinghealth.com/AH-Meat-Mysteries-UncleanAndUnclean-TheHistoryHumanDiet.html (accessed January 21, 2010).

4. Gloria Tsang, "Farm Raised Salmon vs. Wild Salmon," HealthCastle.com, November 2004, http://www.healthcastle.com/wildsalmon-farmraisedsalmon. shtml (accessed January 21, 2010).

5. R. Bromfield, "Honey for Decubitus Ulcers," *Journal of the American Medical Association* 224, no. 6 (1973): 905.

6. "Too Much Honey," Health Benefits of Honey, Honey-health.com/honey-24.shtml (accessed June 7, 2011).

7. Diana Herrington, "7 Tips to Stop Sugar Cravings," Greenwink, Greenwink.net/?p=9290 (accessed June 7, 2011).

CHAPTER FOUR
BEYOND THE PALE

1.Visual Economics, "How Countries Spend Their Money," http://www.visualeconomics.com/how-countries-spend-their-money (accessed June 7, 2011).

2. Thayer & Smith, "The New Testament Greek Lexicon," http://www.studylight.org/lex/grk/view.cgi?number=4982 (accessed June 7, 2011).

3. Why Files, "Minding the Body," www.whyfiles.org/039emotion/coe.html (accessed June 7, 2011).

4. Adam Cohen, "Forgiveness," University of California, Berkeley, Greater Good Science Center, http://greatergood.berkeley.edu/research/research_forgiveness_cohen.html (accessed June 7, 2011).

5. "Forgiveness and Healing," Linktv.org/globalspirit/forgiveness (accessed June 7, 2011).

6. Robert Kolar, "Does God Heal Today?" http://healingscripture.com/ (accessed June 7, 2011).

7. American Cancer Society, "Poor Diet, Lack of Exercise as Lethal as Smoking," Cancer.org, March 9, 2004, http://www.cancer.org/docroot/NWS/content/NWS_2_1x_Were_Killing_Ourselves.asp (accessed February 11, 2010).

CHAPTER FIVE
THE SKINNY ON ARTIFICIAL SWEETENERS

1. Christina R. Whitehouse, Joseph Boullata, and Linda A. McCauley, "The Potential Toxicity of Artificial Sweeteners," *Continuing Education* 56, no. 6 (2008): 254.

2. "Aspartame: What You Don't Know Can Hurt You," http://aspartame.mercola.com/ (accessed June 7, 2011).

3. Christina R. Whitehouse, Joseph Boullata, and Linda A. McCauley, "The Potential Toxicity of Artificial Sweeteners," *Continuing Education* 56, no. 6 (2008): 254.

4. Mercola, "Aspartame: What You Don't Know Can Hurt You," http://aspartame.mercola.com/ (accessed June 7, 2011).

5. Janet Starr Hull, "Dangers of Aspartame Poisoning," Sweetpoison.com/aspartame-information.html (accessed June 7, 2011).

6. Mike Adams, "Interview with Dr. Russell Blaylock on devastating health effects of MSG, aspartame and excitotoxins," NaturalNews.com, September 2006, http://www.naturalnews.com/020550.html (accessed February 11, 2010).

7. Daniel J. DeNoon, "Drink More Diet Soda, Gain More Weight?" WebMD, http://www.webmd.com/diet/news/20050613/drink-more-diet-soda-gain-more-weight (accessed June 7, 2011).

8. MedicineNet, "Artificial Sweeteners," http://www.medicinenet.com/artificial_sweeteners/page5.htm (accessed June 7, 2011).

9. MedicineNet, "Artificial Sweeteners," http://www.medicinenet.com/artificial_sweeteners/page6.htm (accessed June 7, 2011).

10. American Psychological Association, "Artificial Sweeteners Linked To Weight Gain," *ScienceDaily* (2008). Accessed June 7, 2011).

11. MedicineNet, "Artificial Sweeteners," http://www.medicinenet.com/artificial_sweeteners/page5.htm (accessed June 7, 2011).

12. MedicineNet, "Artificial Sweeteners," http://www.medicinenet.com/artificial_sweeteners/page10.htm (accessed June 7, 2011).

13. Center for Science in the Public Interest, "Sample Quotes from Cancer Experts' Letters on Acesulfame Testing," http://www.cspinet.org/reports/asek-quot.html (accessed June 7, 2011).

14. Marcelle Pick, "Sugar substitutes and the potential danger of Splenda," Womentowomen.com/healthyweight/splenda.aspx (accessed June 7, 2011).

15. James Bowen, "The Lethal Science of Splenda—A Poisonous Chlorocarbon," http://www.rense.com/general65/splend.htm (accessed June 7, 2011).

16. Scott Reich, "Sucralose," http://www.drscottreich.com/node/12 (accessed June 7, 2011).

17. Fatsecret.com/diary.aspx?pa=fjrd&rid=1051774 (accessed June 7, 2011).

18. Nayda Rondon, "Xylitol Health Benefits and Potential Side Effects," http://www.yourdentistryguide.com/xylitol/ (accessed June 7, 2011).

19. Oakland Periodontal Associates, "Periodontal Disease," Oaklandperio.com/perio.html (accessed June 7, 2011).

20. http://en.wikipedia.org/wiki/stevia (accessed June 7, 2011).

21. Mark D. Gold, "Current Status of Stevia," Holisticmed.com/sweet/stv-alert.txt (accessed June 7, 2011).

22. Rob McCaleb, quoted at "Stevia Dangers?" Stevia.net, http://www.stevia.net/safety.htm (accessed May 23, 2011).

CHAPTER SIX
CIRCUIT TRAINING

1. Cooperinstitute.org/go/couse_registration/index.cfm?class_id=9049

2. http://en.wikipedia.org/wiki/Dumbbell (accessed June 7, 2011).

3. Robin Lloyd, "The Most Important Exercise Tip," LiveScience.com May 30, 2006, http://www.livescience.com/10490-important-exercise-tip.html (accessed June 7, 2011).

CHAPTER SEVEN
REMEMBER THE SABBATH

1. http://www.jewfaq.org/shabbat.htm (accessed June 7, 2011).

2. Robert Jamieson, A. R. Fausset, and David Brown, *The Commentary, Critical and Explanatory, on the Whole Bible*, s.v. "Hebrews 10:25," available at Biblos.com, http://bible.cc/hebrews/10-25.htm (accessed May 24, 2011).

3. Ibid.

4. "Importance of Sleep: Six Reasons Not to Skimp on Sleep," *The Harvard Women's Health Watch,* Health.harvard.edu, http://www.health.harvard.edu/press_releases/importance_of_sleep_and_health (accessed March 23, 2010).

CHAPTER EIGHT
A MIGHTY MUSCLE

1. "Your Sense of Taste," http://library.thinkquest.org/3750/taste/taste.html (accessed June 7, 2011).

2. Jennifer Stewart, "A Word For Everything," Write 101.com, 2004, http://www.write101.com/W.Tips298.htm (accessed June 7, 2011).

3. Winston Churchill, quoted at ThinkExist.com, http://thinkexist.com/quotation/a_vocabulary_of_truth_and_simplicity_will_be_of/185644.html (accessed May 24, 2011).

4. "RA Connection," *Purdue University Women's Resource Office,* http://www.purdue.edu/wro/raconnection.shtml (accessed May 24, 2011).

CHAPTER NINE
BEYOND FLESH AND BLOOD

1. Rusty Blann, "Victory Over the 'Wiles' of the Devil," *S.O.A.P. for Today* (blog), http://pastorrustysblog.blogspot.com/2008/08/victory-over-wiles-of-devil.html (accessed May 24, 2011).

2. Ibid.

3. Ibid.

4. Ibid.

5. Jeremy D. Myers, "Belt of Truth," http://www.tillhecomes.org/Text_Sermons/Ephesians/Eph6_14a.htm (accessed June 7, 2011).

6. "Bible Literacy Slipping, Experts Say," Southern Nazarene University, http://home.snu.edu/~HCULBERT/literacy.htm (accessed March 19, 2010).

7. Merriam-Webster Dictionary Online, s.v. "righteousness," http://www.merriam-webster.com/dictionary/righteousness (accessed May 24, 2011).

8. Legio VI, "Caligae—Military Boot," Legvi.tripod.com/id84.html (accessed June 7, 2011).

9. Ibid.

10. Frugalsites.net/jesus/crucifixion.htm (accessed June 7, 2011).

11. http://en.wikipedia.org/wiki/Scutum_(shield) (accessed June 7, 2011).

12. Steven A. Austin and Andrew A. Snelling, "Startling Evidence for Noah's Flood,"Answersingenesis.org, December 1992, http://www.answersingenesis.org/creation/v15/i1/flood.asp (accessed March 20, 2010).

13. "Are Students Losing Their Religion on Campus?" ABCNews.go.com, http://abcnews.go.com/GMA/story?id=1375842&page=2 (accessed March 20, 2010).

14. Martin Luther King Jr., quoted at ThinkExist.com, http://thinkexist.com/quotation/faith_is_taking_the_first_step_even_when_you_don/214973.html (accessed May 24, 2011).

15. Bicycle Health Safety Institute, "Helmet Related Statistics From Many Sources," http://www.bhsi.org/stats.htm (accessed June 7, 2011).

16. Chaplain Gordon James Klingenschmitt, "Jesus Christ Banned From Prayer by Pennsylvania House Speaker," Nowpublic.com, July 11, 2009 (accessed March 21, 2010).

17. Godfire.net/TheWord2.html

18. Adam Clarke, *The Adam Clarke Commentary,* available at GodRules.net, http://godrules.net/library/clarke/clarke1joh2.htm (accessed March 22, 2010).

ABOUT THE AUTHOR

DIANA ANDERSON IS a personal trainer and freelance writer whose battle with anorexia as a teen led her closer to God and the power of His Word as she learned to view and honor her body as a temple of the Holy Spirit. Now she is passionate about sharing the message of truly complete fitness—for mind, body, and soul—with young women. She divides her time between Tyler and Austin, Texas.

CONTACT THE AUTHOR

Diana Anderson can be reached at
www.facebook.com/dianaandersoninc.

You can also follow her on Twitter
@dianafit4faith

Subscribe to her blog, **www.dianafit.com**.